Evaluating Hospital-Based Ambulatory Care

Evaluating Hospital-Based Ambulatory Care

A Case Study

William C. Stratmann
The University of Rochester

Ralph Ullman
Columbia University

LexingtonBooks
D.C. Heath and Company
Lexington, Massachuestts
Toronto

To D.M.

Library of Congress Cataloging in Publication Data

Stratmann, William C
 Evaluating hospital-based ambulatory care.

 Includes index.
 1. Genesee Hospital. 2. Genesee Health Service. 3. Hospitals—Outpa-
tient services—Case studies. I. Ullman, Ralph, joint author. II. Title.
[DNLM: 1. Ambulatory care. 2. Outpatient clinics, Hospital. WX205 S899e]
RA982.R6G57   363.1'7   77-11403
ISBN 0-669-02096-6

Published simultaneously in Canada

Printed in the United States of America

International Standard Book Number: 0-669-02096-6

Library of Congress Catalog Card Number: 77-11403

Contents

List of Figures and Tables

Preface and Acknowledgments

The concept of hospital-sponsored primary-care group practice is no longer new, in part because of the efforts of the many people who were involved in the creation of the Genesee Health Service. As an alternative to traditional hospital outpatient clinics, it has become a well-known national prototype. It has provided a stimulus for the creation of larger-scale programs to improve hospital ambulatory care. With financial support from the Robert Wood Johnson Foundation, other community hospitals have been encouraged to construct comparable innovative ambulatory-care facilities. In 1980, under the provisions of Public Law 95-626, federal funding was initiated for the planning, development, and operation of hospital-affiliated primary-care centers directed to medically underserved populations.

Those who participated in the development of the Genesee Health Service can be justifiably proud of their contributions to the improvement of ambulatory-care delivery. We are hopeful that this book will be helpful to those who must assess the usefulness of their own efforts to enhance the well-being of the millions of people who, of necessity, must rely on institutional facilities for their basic health care needs.

Acknowledgments

The research on which this book is based could not have been accomplished without the assistance of many people. We thank James Block, Ronald Press, and Marshall Rozzi, who were instrumental in the development of the Genesee Health Service, for the opportunity to participate in its evaluation and for their ongoing support and encouragement. We also thank Donna Regenstreif for her participation in the early research effort and for her perceptive comments throughout on various aspects of our work. For their patience and cooperation, we express our appreciation to the administration and staff of Genesee Hospital and to all those in the Genesee Health Service who bore the burden of our research. During various stages of the research, we benefited from the advice of Gordon Black, Ned Boatright, Stephen Brown, Arthur Goldberg, Robert Haggerty, David Kotok, Richard McKelvey, Jerry Solon, James Tobin, and William Weller. We also thank our cheerful and efficient research assistants and secretarial staff. The senior author is especially grateful to William Riker and Richard Niemi, and to the University of Rochester for the administrative support that greatly facilitated the preparation of the manuscript.

We are indebted to the Carnegie Corporation of New York for financial support during the earlier research and to the National Library of Medicine (NIH Grant LM00046) for support during the preparation of the manuscript. Although this volume obviously has profited from the help of many people, the authors, of course, are solely responsible for its contents and deficiencies.

1

Research Issues, Concepts, and Strategies

Ten years ago, Genesee Hospital's outpatient clinics and emergency room probably were not much different from those that might have been found at any other urban community hospital. Outpatient areas in these institutions then were described typically as unattractive settings in which patients endure long waits to receive episodic care from rotating teams of harried housestaff and volunteer attendings. Yet, increasing numbers of patients were turning to Genesee for their basic health-care needs. To make matters worse, the hospital annually incurred financial deficits from outpatient operations. It was evident that something had to be done, and after considerable debate the hospital's board approved a set of sweeping changes. All outpatient divisions were to be incorporated in a single department, under the direction of a full-time physician administrator. Planning for the restructuring of the emergency room was begun, so as to make it more responsive to patient demand. The most significant change affected the outpatient clinics, which were replaced by a group practice of full-time, salaried physicians—the Genesee Health Service (GHS).

Since its inception the new health service has become institutionalized as a primary-care unit within the hospital structure. It now provides for the ongoing health-care needs of thousands of people and has successfully integrated the hospital's outpatient population into a socioeconomically mixed practice broadly representative of the community. During its formative years, the authors were responsible for the conduct of an evaluative study of the impact of the new health-care model. This book reports on that research project and attempts to provide the reader with an understanding of how complex changes in hospital-based ambulatory care can be evaluated.

Background for Change at Genesee

Most communities like to think of themselves as unique. Rochester, New York, is no exception. Many people know Rochester as the home of Kodak, the corporate giant founded by George Eastman in the late 1800s. Today Rochester's reputation for innovation in health-care planning and development derives in no small part from the support of Kodak and other local industries. Industry had always been concerned about health-care issues, and the more so in recent years as escalating costs of health-care delivery have

1

increased the cost of employee benefits programs. Although Kodak's health-care benefits are not exceptional by industrial standards, the company has been very generous in lending its executive expertise to the cause of health-care planning. Local leadership has been exercised also by the Industrial Management Council, the University of Rochester's School of Medicine and Dentistry, and a succession of public and private organizations.

More than forty years ago, six local hospitals formed the Rochester Hospital Council in an effort to coordinate the planning of the city's institutional needs. Now called the Rochester Regional Hospital Association, the organization's jurisdiction has been expanded to include a ten-county area. The early initiatives of local hospitals have been complemented over the years by community organizations such as the Health Council of Monroe County. In 1968, at about the same time that the concept of federally supported regional planning was being formalized, a committee of the Health Council was engaged in a study of the health-care needs of inner-city people. Their report recommended that consideration be given to the creation of a network of inner-city health-care facilities, and federal funds were obtained to organize a non-profit corporation, Neighborhood Health Centers of Monroe County, Inc. (NHC), which then assumed the task of planning the development of a network of health-care centers for the inner city.

At about the same time, the administrators and medical staff of the Genesee Hospital, a 400-bed community institution established before the turn of the century, had begun an independent assessment of their responsibilities for providing primary care in the form of outpatient services.[1] A newly appointed assistant director was assigned the responsibility for outpatient planning, but the administration was handicapped by a lack of financial resources and by a lack of consensus among the medical staff as to what improvements should be made. The debate continued through the summer of 1969 with little progress toward a solution. In the fall of that year a significant event occurred. The administration learned of a new program in the Office of Economic Opportunity (OEO) that was directed at the planning and development of inner-city health-care facilities. News of the program also quickly spread through the community.

Its historical reputation for successful innovation in health-care planning made Rochester a viable candidate for support. A major issue was how such support should be sought. Some thought that the regional planning agency should take the initiative in preparing a grant application to OEO. But inner-city community groups had other ideas. To them the regional planning agency was "establishment." Inner-city groups traditionally have differed among themselves about many matters. The issue of health care, however, transcended petty jealousies. If federal funds were to be applied for, they wanted to be a part of the process. In a letter to the planning agency, the leader of the city-wide coalition of community groups expressed the view that the planning agency could not serve the purposes of inner-city people as well as could the newly formed NHC organization. Soon thereafter the NHC board began to reflect much greater inner-city representation, as community groups took positive steps to ensure their input into the planning process. The lesson was not lost on Genesse's planners. They effected close coordination with NHC and with Genesee's own patient constituency, who were represented by a community group known as the Southeast Area Coalition (SEAC). In the ensuing months, Genesee's planners worked in collaboration with SEAC's health-care task force, to the mutual benefit of both organizations.

Genesee Hospital's initial response to OEO's solicitation for proposals outlined briefly the goal of eliminating the separate system of care for clinic patients by the creation of a new ambulatory-care center in the hospital's professional building. The new program would be housed in an attractive facility and would strive to achieve much the same appeal as that which characterized private sources of health care. As planning continued, it became obvious that Genesee's contribution to the developing plan for a network of centers would represent a radical departure from tradition. By the spring of 1971, as the network proposal neared completion, some members of the medical community were expressing strong opposition to the project. They voiced concern "that the clinics would destroy the private practice of medicine by serving the well-to-do as well as the poor,"[2] and argued "that the clinics would be more expensive than visits to doctor's offices, would provide inferior medical care and would be short-staffed or staffed by 'transient' doctors."[3] Yet, opposition notwithstanding, a special committee of the Medical Society reported general endorsement of the network proposal, reflecting the consensual view that the centers *did* offer the prospect of improved health care for inner-city people.

The results of the very difficult planning efforts culminated in April 1971 with the submission by NHC of a comprehensive proposal for the creation of three new community health centers. Although each of these was to be associated with a community hospital, only the center at Genesee would result in the closing of a traditional outpatient clinic. The other two new centers would be "free-standing." Together with two existing centers, a network of facilities was created that encircled the inner-city area. The grant, which was approved for funding by OEO in July 1971, differed from customary OEO grants in several important ways. First, there were no geographic boundaries to the service areas of the proposed centers; second, subsidization of care was given the marginally poor; third, the 20 percent limitation of the proportion of nonpoor who could be served was removed; and, fourth, centers were to be located in so-called transition zones, making them readily accessibly to people with different socioeconomic backgrounds. Collectively, these provisos reflected the firm belief of planners that the success of efforts to improve care for inner-city residents necessitated that new facilities appeal to all socioeconomic groups. "Health care provided exclusively for the poor," they argued, "will become poor care."[4]

Federal approval of funds for the network allowed Genesee's administrators to attack many of the deficiencies in hospital outpatient care that had been observed and discussed nationally. The typical outpatient department existed usually as a collection of specialty clinics in which medical services were provided in a piecemeal fashion, either through training programs or by physicians who contributed small portions of their time. The absence of any single physician to assume the continuing management of patients was viewed as a significant deterrent to good health care. By employing full-time, salaried physicians, GHS would be designed to provide medical care with accessibility and continuity, thereby to attain increased patient satisfaction, improved compliance, and more attention to measures of prevention.

Initial plans were for the center to consist of three family-oriented teams of health workers. Each team would include two internists, two pediatricians, one obstetrician/gynecologist, a nurse or nurse practitioner, a public health nurse, and several family health workers. Access to specialist services also would be provided, and dental services were located immediately adjacent. In sum, a complete range of services were to be made available.

Although not restricted by geographic boundaries, GHS was expected to appeal primarily to a natural service constituency in the southeast section of the city. The potential patient population was estimated at about forty-five thousand people, about eight thousand of whom were defined as medically indigent. An ambulatory services board consisting of twenty-one members would be established to oversee the operation. A majority would be patient-consumers, and the remainder would represent the hospital's board of governors (to which the ambulatory services board would function in an advisory capacity), administrative staff, and medical staff. It was hoped that the new center would become financially viable in three years.

Research Strategy

Genesee's planners thought they understood the hospital's outpatient population and the broader community to which they sought to appeal. They knew that the success of their venture would depend on the validity of their perceptions about what people wanted in the form of health-care services. Moreover, they viewed Rochester as a microcosm of our larger health-care system. They believed that the practice of medicine in Rochester and the norms of patient and provider behavior that prevailed there probably were little different from those elsewhere. They reasoned that, if their assumptions were correct, the Genesee Health Service might have wide application as a prototype for change in other urban hospital-based ambulatory-care settings. It seemed worthwhile therefore to attempt to document the process of change at Genesee, and to assess the extent to which the new service achieved the objectives of its designers. To this end they sought and received a foundation grant to create an evaluation unit within the hospital's newly formed Department of Ambulatory Services, in which the Genesee Health Service was to become an integral component.

Although familiar with techniques of basic research, the authors had little background in health services. This lack necessitated that we assimilate a great deal of information in a relatively short period of time. Extensive discussions were held with health-service planners. Research assistants were hired and assigned the task of gleaning from the health-care literature a bibliography suitable for our needs. A library of reference materials quickly was collected, abstracted, and indexed. We also availed ourselves of the advice of several outside consultants. We were frustrated by the need for haste, and yet inhibited from getting too involved in the details of a research design before we had completed a survey of the existing literature. Gradually, all too slowly it seemed at the time, we began to integrate our basic research ideas with those of others who already had broken ground in the field. We thus formulated the framework for our research design.

As a "given," we knew that the goal of the health service was to provide "good" or "better" health care for a specific population, the users of the hospital's outpatient clinics and emergency room. But the new service also was being designed to appeal to a much broader community of users. Clearly needed were criteria that might be used to define the dependent variable *health-care delivery*, and to conceive of appropriate standards by which the new service could be assessed, with respect to these criteria. We hoped also that our study of the Genesee Health Service would enhance our understanding of the general process of health-care utilization. We wanted to develop a theoretical explanation of this process, and to develop a methodology that would permit planners elsewhere to assess the value of proposed changes in their own institutional settings. It seemed to us that, in the final analysis, the utility of the care facility at Genesee, or of any such facility elsewhere, ought best to be judged by the extent to which it is accepted by the patient population for whom it is designed. Acceptance, as such, can readily be measured by use. The essence of our research design is the posited assumption that patient utilization of any ambulatory-care facility is a *behavioral phenomenon*.

Rational-Choice Theory

One of the things that seems to distinguish man from other creatures on our planet is his ability to reason—to think, to calculate, and to make decisions. Human behavior can, in the main, be characterized as the identification, ordering, and pursuit of goals. Typically, human behavior seems to effect the most logical and efficient means toward achieving these goals, given the individual's understanding of the circumstances related to his actions. Economists describe the behavior of economic man as rational if his behavior appears to be efficient. Thus, in the marketplace, firms seek to maximize profits while consumers seek to maximize utility. With these ends posited, economic man is assumed to use the most efficient means to achieve them, and efficiency is maximized at the point of the least input of scarce resources necessary to achieve a given goal. This economic framework of rationality has been extended to other disciplines. In a classic work, Anthony Downs creates a concept of political man as an analogue of economic man.[5] According to Downs, political parties seek to maximize political power, while voters seek to maximize political utility. The voting act is the process by which an individual differentiates among alternatives on the basis of expected political benefits. Rational behavior is manifested if a voter calculates logically the benefits that alternative candidates might be expected to yield, and then opts for the candidate whom he thinks will yield him the greatest satisfaction.

The value of these applications of rational-choice theory is the contribution they make to our understanding of human behavior. They afford causal explanations that permit us to anticipate future events with a high degree of predictive efficacy. The circumstances in which the basic theory can be applied are those in which the phenomena to be explained involves human choice.[6] We viewed patient utilization of ambulatory services as the manifestation of such a choice process. Hence, we thought that the theory of rational choice could readily be adapted to the study of the new ambulatory-care facility.

On Choosing a Source of Care

The assumption that most human behavior is purposefully oriented and that people generally seem able to perceive needs or goals relative to which their behavior can be described is the foundation of our research design.[7]

We postulate that people can identify their health-related needs or goals and that their utilization of health-care sources is a manifestation of their purposeful movement toward these goals. Our discussion of needs and goals and of the means by which these might be achieved suggests the use of some sort of scale by which we might measure the utility of the options open to the decision-maker. By utility we mean the perceived usefulness of the need, goal, or option. Clearly some things are more important than others. It follows that people should be able to differentiate among the factors that relate to a decision as a function of their relative importance. For example, to a prospective car buyer such things as gas mileage, size, speed, horsepower, color, comfort, or maintenance might be logical elements in his decision. For lack of a better term we call these elements *decision-components*. We assume that an individual can order these with respect to their relative importance to his choice of automobile. Further, we assume that an individual can distinguish among alternative automobiles with respect to these decision-components as a function of expected satisfaction. Finally, we assume that in some cognitive or subconscious way people calculate the overall utility to them of each alternative automobile, and that this calculation involves the relative importance of decision-components, and the expected satisfaction that each car will yield with respect to each decision-component. Thus, we argue that the car buyer uses this type of rational calculus to effect his decision. We believe that by some similar calculus the prospective consumer of health services makes a decision to use a particular source of care. We reasoned that the study of this decision-making process would yield a set of criteria that could be used to evaluate a new program.

Evaluating the Changes at Genesee

It was quite clear to us that GHS would not achieve success easily. A quality program of primary-care delivery involves much more than architecturally pleasing surroundings. Among other things, continuity of care normally requires full-time physicians. To recruit a competent and motivated staff, the new service would have to offer the same type of professional challenges that could be found in a private group practice. The planners also were aware of the outpatient department's annual deficits. They realized that if GHS was to be financially viable, it would have to generate a large portion of its revenues from middle-class, fee-for-service patients. In short, the success of the Genesee Health Service would depend greatly on its appeal to a broad segment of the Rochester community. We concluded, therefore, that our assessment of the new care program would have to involve the application of community-wide standards of care delivery. Accordingly, we had to derive from rational-choice theory a model of patient behavior that would permit us to identify criteria that consumers use to select a source of ambulatory-care delivery.

Two antithetical assumptions underlie opposing views of the wisdom of patient behavior. Some people believe that patients are incapable of choosing wisely from among different kinds of health services the one that can best serve their individual needs, or even of knowing what those needs are. Alternatively, other people believe that patients do understand their needs and how best to achieve them.[8] We think it useful to view the fulfillment of individual needs as a causal process that, for purposes of study, can be broken down logically into a sequence of decisions that are triggered by the recognition of a medical problem:

Does the perceived need warrant medical care?

If so, what kind of care is required?

Is the potential benefit of such care greater than the cost of time, money, or whatever that may be involved in obtaining that care?

How do the costs and the benefits associated with the option to seek care compare with cost-benefit assessments of other competing needs such as food, clothing, shelter, or whatever?

Finally, if the decision is made to obtain medical care, which facility from among those available seems most likely to meet the individual's standards?

We saw a clear relationship between the process by which people select an ambulatory-care facility and our task of evaluating GHS. We knew that a variety of factors influenced that patient's choice of source of care. We reasoned that, if we could identify and define objectively the components of the patient's decision, we would have established a set of valid criteria with which to evaluate patient satisfaction.

With the acceptance of the general strategy for defining the dependent variable *health-care delivery*, we were able to complete our research design. We would need to develop an extensive open-ended protocol for use in a community-wide survey of households in the Rochester area. We recognized the need to control for a variety of variables that were antecedent to the process of choosing a source of care, for example the perceived severity or urgency of the presenting problem that makes access to care a necessity. We also would have to differentiate between the choice of care for a child, and that for an adult. Comparable survey instruments would later be used to interview Genesee Health Service patients, and to elicit their opinion about the new program. These surveys also would attempt to document a respondent's utilization of services. While we had no reason to question the reliability of reported utilization, we saw the need for more precise documentation, particularly with respect to the population that used Genesee's clinics and emergency room.

In surveying the literature on hospital utilization we found that, although planners speak in familiar terms of their institution's patient population, little is actually known about these patients. Facilities are designed and staffed to meet patient demand, usually measured in terms of *visits*. Medical care in this setting has little continuity and remains essentially episodic and crisis-oriented. Under such circumstances, there is slight incentive to acquire more detailed information. As we explain later, although the task of describing accurately the hospital's outpatient population and its utilization of hospital services proved a challenging task in itself, we needed this information in order to evaluate any changes in utilization at Genesee. For example, it was hoped that use of the emergency room would be reduced once GHS became operational and former clinic patients became accustomed to relying on the new facility for their health-care needs. We needed to acquire appropriate data with which to test this hypothesis.

Although the study of patient attitudes about health care, the measurement of criteria for evaluation, and the documentation of actual patient utilization were expected to consume most of our time and resources, another issue also merited attention. We were interested in examining the financial impact that the new service would have on the hospital and on the provision of care more generally. To do so we would have to face not only the complexities of hospital finance, but also the requirement for detailed longitudinal information.

In the following chapters we present our analysis of community attitudes about ambulatory-care delivery, an explanation of patient utilization of ambulatory-care services at Genesee, a description of the former outpatient clinics and the new health service, an assessment of the impact of GHS, patients' perceptions of GHS, and some concluding comments.

Notes

1. For an anthropologist's view of this planning process see Donna I. Regenstreif, "Innovation in Hospital-Based Ambulatory Care: Some Sources, Patterns, and Implications of Change," *Human Organization* 36(1977) :43.

2. *Rochester Times Union*, March 17, 1971, p. B1.

3. Ibid.

4. Neighborhood Health Centers of Monroe County, Inc., "Prelim-

inary Proposal for a Community Health Network," Rochester, N.Y., January 1971.

5. Anthony Downs, *An Economic Theory of Democracy* (New York: Harper and Row, 1957).

6. For an explanation of its application to the voting act see William C. Stratmann, "The Calculus of Rational Choice," *Public Choice* 17(1974) :93.

7. This concept was first presented in William C. Stratmann, "A Model for Evaluating Ambulatory Services at a Community Hospital," (Paper delivered at the 69th Annual Meeting of the American Public Health Association, San Francisco, November 1973.) A more extensive discussion is available in William C. Stratmann, "A Study of Community Attitudes About Health Care: The Delivery of Ambulatory Services," *Medical Care* 13 (1975) :537.

8. William C. Richardson and Duncan Neuhauser, "First Question in Health Planning: Does the Public Know What It Wants or Not?" *Modern Hospital* 110(1968) :115.

2

Attitudes about Ambulatory-Care Delivery

In our explanation of the rationale for our research strategy, we suggest that the patient's choice of an ambulatory-care facility is not unlike many other consumer decisions. Every consumer product or service has associated with it a set of categorical attributes, which vary in importance depending on individual values, beliefs, and attitudes. We believe that the consumer judges the utility of alternative products or services with respect to these attributes, which we define as decision-components. We believe that people, at least subconciously, rank-order these decision-components in accord with their relative importance. When confronted with the need to make a choice, they integrate the importance of these factors with information about their alternatives and by some unknown but rational calculus derive a preference for one alternative or another. We do not suggest that people actually sit down and perform these calculations. What matters is that people act as though they make their choices in this way. This notion is the basis for theories of rational choice. As with the person who buys an automobile, so with the health-services consumer. Health-service facilities exist to serve the needs of patients. In the final analysis the utilization of health care is a function of patient satisfaction with the process and outcome of care. We reasoned that the extent to which the Genesee Health Service met the goals of its designers should be a function of the manner in which it would be received by its target population. We also reasoned that the criteria that patients use to make this judgment would be equally appropriate for our evaluation of the new service.

In designing the study of community attitudes about health care, we had several objectives. As with the concomitant study of patient utilization of the outpatient clinics and emergency room, we needed to establish baseline information. We wanted later to be able to compare attitudes of GHS patients with attitudes of the community as a whole, thereby to test the intended broad appeal of the new program. In fulfilling this objective, we wanted to control for the urgency of the medical problem that makes a trip to a health-care facility necessary. Thus, we wanted to find out whether the criteria that respondents use to judge a facility varies, depending on the

Material in this chapter has been adapted from William C. Stratmann, "A Study of Consumer Attitudes About Health Care: The Delivery of Ambulatory Services," *Medical Care* 13(1975) :537; and William C. Stratmann and Ralph Ullman, "A Study of Community Attitudes About Health Care: The Role of the Emergency Room," *Medical Care* 13(1975) :1033. Used with permission.

perceived urgency of the medical need. For similar reasons, we thought it important to ask parents to distinguish between the criteria that they use to select a facility for themselves, and those that they use to select a source of care for their children.

The need to conduct the survey about health-care attitudes also offered heuristic opportunities. It permitted us to apply rational-choice theory to the context of patient use of health services. From reported respondent attitudes about health care, we should be able to predict the type of facility that the person would be most likely to use, depending on the nature of the patient's presenting problem. A high degree of predictive efficacy would tend to substantiate the validity of our model of patient behavior. Further, the survey permitted us to investigate the relationship between sociodemographic variables and utilization of health care services. Although patient behavior has been attributed to individual sociodemographic characteristics, we do not believe that such characteristics are causal determinants of behavior. Actions result from cognitive thought, not because of sex, or age, or race. Thus, while observed associations between sociodemographic characteristics and patterns of utilization can be used to describe a patient population, we do not believe they explain the behavior of this population. Finally, we hoped to be able to compare patient attitudes about health care with physician attitudes on this subject. To this end we planned to field a mail survey among physicians with questions based on the survey of community attitudes.

Survey Methods

From an area with a population of approximately 580,000 we selected randomly 50 percent of the census tracts. Cluster sampling proportional to the population of each selected tract ultimately yielded a sample of 437 households. An additional eighty-four households were selected randomly from characteristically low-income census tracts. A professional staff conducted in-the-home interviews with heads of households. Interviews lasted about two hours. See the appendix for the complete protocol.

The survey instrument was designed to elicit from the respondent his health-care history and attitudes about ambulatory-care utilization. Respondents were asked first to identify their central source of care with the following question:[1] "Is there any one place or person that you feel you can rely upon when you need help about a medical problem? Is there someone or some place that you feel you can always turn to when you need medical help or advice?" If the respondent replied in the affirmative, he was asked whether it would involve going to a hospital emergency room, a hospital clinic, a private doctor's ofice, a clinic at work, or a neighborhood health center. Assuming the nonavailability of his central source, the respondent was asked to identify from the list of alternatives a substitute source to which he would go under those circumstances. The respondent was then asked a series of questions about each of the five types. We wanted to find out where people went for care, why they used a specific source of care, and how they felt about the treatment they received. We asked: Have you ever gone to a _____? Why haven't you ever gone to a _____? Which one (s) wouldn't you go to again? Why? What was it that first made you decide to go there rather than some place else? What do you like about _____? What do you dislike about _____? The answers to these questions were recorded verbatim by the interviewer and later were used by coders to define the criteria that respondents used to distinguish their feelings.

Respondents were asked to define the medical problems that prompted their use of different facilities: When you go to a _____, is the problem usually so urgent that you have to see a doctor right away, or can you usually wait a while and put off seeing him until the next day? Finally, for different types of problems respondents were asked to estimate their total number of visits during the past year. Similar questions were asked of parents with regard to where they took their children for medical care and why. Additional questions were asked to ascertain respondent views about the accessibility of health care at night and on weekends, about waiting time, about annoying incidents that may have occurred during a visit, and about what they thought were the more important health-care issues that confronted the American people.

The questionnaire was very demanding of the respondent. Of interest, contrary to our intial apprehension about the length of the questionnaire, we found that most people were quite willing to discuss at length their personal health experiences. In some instances interviewers found it very difficult to complete the questionnaire within a reasonable period of time. Interviewers were able to document from the responses to the series of open-ended questions a rich description of respondent attitudes, from which we eventually distilled a large universe of evaluative criteria.

The Calculus of Rational Choice

Our earlier conceptualization of rational choice led us to posit the following assumptions:

1. A person can identify the factors that constitute the components of his decision to select a source of ambulatory care.
2. A person can order and value these components in a consistent manner.

3. A person can evaluate alternative health facilities relative to these decision-components.

Given this set of assumptions, we hypothesized that a patient should use most often the facility that appears to offer the greatest overall utility.

Operationalizing the calculation of a respondent's rational choice proved time-consuming. During the course of the interview, evaluative criteria were listed on a card by the interviewer. When all open-ended questions had been answered, the respondent was handed the card and asked to rank-order each of the listed criteria. The procedure involved a series of paired comparisons. The respondent was asked to identify the most important criterion, to which the interviewer assigned a value of ten. Using a ten-point scale the respondent then was asked to assign a value to his second-most important criterion. Subsequent paired comparisons followed until all criteria had been assigned values of importance. Then the respondent was asked to evaluate each of the five different types of health-care source with respect to each criterion, again using a ten-point scale. Later, using a simple algorithm, we calculated the respondent's *rational choice*—the type of facility that had the greatest overall utility.[2]

Our methodology may appear to be unnecessarily complicated. Any simple seven- or nine-point scale would be adequate for the analysis of an *individual's* decision-components. However, a methodological cul-de-sac occurs if we aggregate these characteristically ordinal values to compare individual attitudes. Manifestly, the aggregation of these ordinal data is an interpersonal comparison of subjective measures of utility. Hence, we must view these data with skepticism.[3]

We cannot assume that the utility of a particular numerical value that one person assigns to the importance of, say, quality of care, represents the same utility to another person who might assign the factor the same scale value, because we do not know how each person perceives the scale itself. However, if we normalize all the scale values that each person assigns to his respective set of decision-components, the measure of individual attitude is grounded no longer on a subjectively perceived scale, but on a decisional situation common to each person. In effect, by normalizing the values that each person assigns to the relative importance of each decision-component in his set, we generate a nonsubjective ratio scale. By summing the set of values and dividing each by the sum of the whole, we obtain as a percentage the *relative* importance of each component to the overall decision. Since the sum of each person's set of component weightings equals 100 percent, we can compare each person's weighting of the importance of a given factor to another person's weighting of the same factor, and a valid measure of their comparative relative importance results. These normalized weighted values of individual decision-components thereby are a function of both the scale value initally assigned and the number of elements that comprise that person's set of decision-components. The multiplication of each of the weighted decision-components by a measure of the respective satisfaction that a person expects from each facility enables the generation of a weighted summation of that person's preferences for alternative facilities, circumvents the problem of interpersonal comparison of utility, and makes possible a meaningful comparative analysis of decisional criteria.[4]

Categories of Criteria

Our application of rational-choice theory is based on a concept of personal utility. To facilitate our analysis of the survey data, we arbitrarily grouped the universe of reported criteria into five categories:

1. Economic factors, such as the cost of services, payment schedule, loss of income incurred by the visit, the availability of free medicine, and the willingness of the provider to accept one insurance program or another.
2. Temporal factors, such as waiting for the doctor, waiting for test results, efficiency of services generally, length of consultation time, and the necessity of subsequent visits.
3. Convenience factors, such as the availability of the doctor, house calls, special services, facilities for food, parking facilities, playroom facilities, emergency appointments, elevators, after-hour appointments, and the location of the health service.
4. Sociopsychological factors, such as the doctor's manner, charitable service, moral principles, ethics, dependability, honesty, courtesy, consideration, sex, staff manner, age, helpfulness, appearance of the facility, patient/doctor relationship, religious affiliation, language spoken, atmosphere of the facility, cleanliness, staff continuity, ethnic identity of personnel, equality of treatment for all people, condescending attitude of staff, privacy for patients, and the socioeconomic characteristics of the other patients.
5. Quality factors, such as the doctor's familiarity with medical history, doctor's competence, qualifications, explanation of problem, staff capability, size, equipment available, specialists available, family orientation, thoroughness of examination, medical treatment, quality of service in general, telephone access to doctor, seeing the same doctor each visit, whether the doctor appeared to take sufficient time with the patient, familiarity of the doctor with latest techniques, and his willingness to refer to specialists.

Each respondent's assigned values were normalized in order to assess

Table 2-1
Aggregated Relative Importance of Decision-Components

	Economic	Temporal	Convenience	Sociopsychological	Quality
Mean normalized weightings	3.6%	11.3%	20.6%	19.7%	44.7%
Standard deviation	(8.4)	(13.9)	(17.2)	(17.2)	(21.2)
Range of weightings	0-44.4%	0-63.0%	0-74.3%	0-76.9%	0-100%
Percentage identifying criterion	17%	46%	70%	68%	97%

their relative importance to the choice of care source and aggregated for the entire population (see table 2-l). Given public concern about the costs of health care,[5] we were surprised to see that respondents perceived economic factors with so little importance until we realized that there is relatively little variance in the customary fees charged by local physicians for office visits. We suspect that cost considerations are much more important to an antecedent decision in the behavioral process of health-care utilization — *whether* care should be sought.

It is apparent from the data that, while technical quality of care is the most important single category, other criteria, collectively, are of greater importance to individual decisions. This seemingly anomalous public perspective of the parameters of the choice of a source of care makes sense when we realize that generally high standards are believed to characterize the care available at almost any facility. Judging from the results of a then current poll of public confidence in that nation's key institutions, in which 57 percent of a national sample accorded to the medical profession "a great deal of confidence," a percentage one-third higher than any other institution named, at the time of the survey people generally did seem satisfied with the American medical-care "system."[6] If a person believes that high standards and quality characterize any service facility, logically, he should perceive other factors as more important, if he must discriminate among these types of services.

Patterns of Preference Weightings

Table 2-2 illustrates the relationship that we discovered between patterns of preference weightings and the sources of care used most often. As expected, economic criteria are less important to those who use private physicians. Apart from this distinction, the two most different overall perspectives are those of emergency-room and neighborhood-health-center users, with respect primarily to convenience and sociopsychological criteria. Those who

Table 2-2
Relationship of Decision-Components to Patterns of Utilization

Facility Used Most	Criterion						
	Economic (%)	Temporal (%)	Convenience (%)	Sociopsychological (%)	Quality (%)	N[a] (%)	No.
Hospital emergency room	7.0	11.4	29.2	9.9	41.8	100	(7)
Hospital clinic	7.2	14.1	12.7	20.8	45.2	100	(40)
Private doctor	2.6	11.4	20.2	20.5	45.3	100	(320)
Clinic at work	7.7	13.0	19.0	16.1	44.2	100	(26)
Neighborhood health center	8.4	9.5	10.6	27.2	44.3	100	(15)
Total sample	3.6	11.3	20.6	19.7	44.7	100	(408)
	< .001[b]	N.S.	< .01	N.S	N.S.		

Source: William C. Stratmann, "A Study of Community Attitudes About Health Care: The Delivery of Ambulatory Services," *Medical Care* 13(1975) :537. With permission.
N.S. = not significant.
[a]These data and the data contained in table 2-3 are based on an enlarged sampling, which included a disproportionately greater number of low-income households. The unweighted distribution by source of care was as follows: Hospital emergency room, 1 percent; Hospital clinic, 7 percent; Private doctor, 84 percent; Clinic at work, 7 percent; and Neighborhood health center, 1 percent.
[b]The significance levels reported relate to the F ratios of between-group means to within-group means in one-way analysis of variance tests, in which the independent row variables are viewed as different "treatment" on the overall mean of the population. t tests of between-group means were also performed because the ANOVA involved unequal cell sizes. These tests support the cited significance levels.

use emergency rooms emphasize the value of convenience and de-emphasize the importance of sociopsychological factors. Among neighborhood health-center users, the reverse is true. The greater importance of socio-psychological factors to the latter group is probably another indication of the responsiveness of this form of care to the indigent and marginally poor,[7] who may resent the impersonal treatment they receive in other settings. People who use hospital clinics share the view of those who use neighborhood health centers with respect to the lesser importance of convenience factors. It is apparent that patients of private physicians assert an attitude somewhere in between emergency-room users and neighborhood-health-center users with respect to both convenience and sociopsychological criteria.

Sociodemographic Characteristics

We discuss earlier our disagreement with a causal interpretation of observed association between sociodemographic characteristics and behavior. Specifically, we argue that individual health-care utilization cannot be explained in this way. Table 2-3 presents the relationship between sociodemographic characteristics and criteria weightings. Although some associations are apparent, in most instances the observed differences in criteria weightings are not significant.

Table 2-4 summarizes the sociodemographic characteristics that appear most likely to be associated with high or low weightings of decisional criteria. It should be noted that this summary identifies only those characteristics most likely to be associated with either high or low criterion weightings. We do not imply that all people with these characteristics hold the same set of perceptions. Similarly, although certain characteristics may appear to correlate with particular utilization patterns, many exceptions to these patterns are evident, particularly among the more heterogeneous suburban subsample.

Table 2-3
Relationship between Decision-Components and Selected
Sociodemographic Characteristics

Sociodemographic Characteristics	Criterion					N	
	Economic (%)	Temporal (%)	Convenience (%)	Sociopsychological (%)	Quality (%)	(%)	No.
Total sample	3.8	11.4	19.8	20.7	44.3	100	(510)
Sex							
Male	4.8	12.0	22.6	15.8	44.7	100	(187)
Female	3.2	11.0	18.1	23.5	44.0	100	(323)
	<.05	N.S.	<.005	<.001	N.S.		
Age							
18-25	3.6	14.2	21.5	20.2	40.5	100	(56)
26-35	4.4	10.9	20.7	21.3	42.6	100	(126)
36-45	3.3	10.4	20.6	22.6	43.1	100	(90)
46-55	3.1	11.7	18.3	18.7	48.2	100	(83)
56-65	5.1	12.4	17.5	20.1	45.0	100	(75)
>65	3.4	10.8	20.5	21.1	44.2	100	(75)
	N.S.	N.S.	N.S.	N.S.	<.001		
Race							
White	3.7	11.1	20.4	20.2	44.6	100	(414)
Black	4.3	12.8	16.3	23.5	43.0	100	(94)
	N.S.	N.S.	.01	N.S.	N.S.		
Education							
≤8 grade	5.1	11.6	16.7	23.2	43.4	100	(87)
>8, ≤12 grade	4.2	11.8	19.9	19.9	44.3	100	(243)
>12 grade	2.7	10.8	21.2	20.5	44.7	100	(180)
	N.S.	N.S.	N.S.	N.S.	N.S.		
Household income							
<$5,000	4.1	13.1	17.0	26.4	39.3	100	(66)
5,000-10,000	5.9	12.1	18.9	19.5	43.6	100	(93)
10,000-15,000	3.6	11.9	20.2	18.4	46.0	100	(140)
15,000-20,000	3.0	9.9	21.2	22.2	43.8	100	(86)
>20,000	2.5	10.4	22.8	17.8	46.6	100	(65)
	N.S.	N.S.	N.S.	<.02	N.S.		

Table 2-3 (continued)

Sociodemographic Characteristics	*Criterion* Economic (%)	Temporal (%)	Convenience (%)	Sociopsychological (%)	Quality (%)	*N* (%)	*No.*
Religion							
Protestant	2.9	12.5	18.9	20.2	45.5	100	(238)
Catholic	4.2	10.5	20.8	20.4	44.1	100	(214)
Jewish	2.7	8.4	22.7	17.8	48.4	100	(10)
Other	5.1	8.9	17.8	28.9	39.2	100	(33)
	< .01	N.S.	N.S.	N.S.	N.S.		
Health status							
Excellent	2.6	10.7	22.1	19.7	44.9	100	(168)
Good	4.4	11.3	20.0	20.3	44.1	100	(210)
Fair	5.0	13.3	18.2	21.0	42.5	100	(100)
Poor	3.0	9.2	11.1	27.4	49.2	100	(29)
	N.S.	N.S.	< .02	N.S.	N.S.		
Insurance							
Medicaid	5.2	15.1	14.9	27.3	37.6	100	(47)
Blue Cross/ Blue Shield	3.6	11.2	19.7	19.9	45.6	100	(339)
Commercial	1.8	9.3	32.8	16.5	39.7	100	(28)
	N.S.	N.S.	< .001	< .02	N.S.		

Source: William C. Stratmann, "A Study of Community Attitudes About Health Care: The Delivery of Ambulatory Services," *Medical Care* 13 (1975):537. With permission.

Note: The sample (N = 510) includes respondents who did not report any actual utilization and, therefore, is larger than the sample reported in the preceding table. N.S. = not significant.

The Test of Rational Choice

With the assistance of a computer, it was relatively simple to calculate each respondent's *rational choice* from his expressed values of criteria importance and, with respect to these criteria, his assessment of alternative sources of care. Given our earlier assumptions about patient behavior, we hypothesized that a person should use most often this type of facility.

We recognize that some people might encounter difficulty in deciding which source to use if they are relatively indifferent in their expected satisfaction from two or more preferred alternatives. We assume that this would have a stochastic effect on their decision-making process, which would be revealed by nearly equal calculated weightings for these facilities, and should be manifested behaviorally by a utilization pattern that favors one or the other of the facilities. For example, if a person anticipates equal satisfaction from two kinds of facility along, say, four of a set of five decision-components, and perceives almost equal satisfaction with respect to the fifth decision-component, then the calculated products of importance and satisfaction when summed for each facility will be only incrementally different. We reason that in such a circumstance the person is likely to

Table 2-4
Summary of Relationship between Sociodemographic Characteristics and Criteria Weightings

Criterion	Low Salience To Those:	High Salience To Those:
Economic	in excellent health, and/or Jewish, college education, greater than $20,000 income, white, female, commercial insurance subscriber, ages 46-55	in fair health, and/or secular religious views, little education, $5-10,000 income, black, male, Medicaid recipient, ages 56-65
Temporal	in excellent health, and/or Catholic, college education, $15-20,000 income, white, female, commercial insurance subscriber, ages 36-45	in fair health, and/or Protestant, high school education, less than $5,000 income, black, male, Medicaid recipient, ages 18-25
Convenience	in poor health, and/or secular religious views, little education, less than $5,000 income, black, female, Medicaid recipient, ages 56-65	in excellent health, and/or Jewish, college education, greater than $20,000 income, white, male, commercial insurance subscriber, ages 18-25
Sociopsychological	in excellent health, and/or Jewish, high school education, $10,-15,000 income, white, male, commercial insurance subscriber, ages 46-55	in poor health, and/or little education, less than $5,000 income, black, female, Medicaid recipient, ages 36-45
Quality	in fair health, and/or secular religious views, little education, less than $5,000 income, black, female, Medicaid recipient, ages 18-25	in poor health, and/or Jewish, college education, greater than $20,000 income, white, male, Blue Cross/Blue Shield subscriber, ages 46-55

choose between the two sources randomly, rather than on the basis of the fixed rule we have posited.

In designing the survey, we reasoned that we could test the reliability of response by comparing the generated weighted preferences for facilities with individual patterns of utilization. Accordingly, we asked the respondents to estimate the frequency with which they used each of the five sources of care. The reported utilization data appear reasonably valid. For example, an average of 5.5 ambulatory visits were reported for the twelve-month period preceding the survey, an acceptable figure when judged against nation-wide data. Further, reported visits to local hospital emergency rooms afforded an estimate of total hospital emergency-room utilization in the Rochester area that was within 10 percent of documented statistics. We conclude that, since the sample data afford reasonably correct estimates of actual utilization, either respondent recall was fairly accurate, or that errors in reporting were random.

Thirteen people in the sample were unable to articulate any cognitive decisional criteria whatsoever. Twenty-five additional individuals were unable either to rank-order decision-components or to evaluate alternative facilities, or were dropped from the sample because the calculation of their weighted preferences involved an invalid utility criterion. For example, a decision-component that represents a circumstance over which the respondent had no control, such as the death or dislocation of a provider, is a reasonable explanation for discontinuing a previous source of care but does not afford an insight into why a patient perceived a present source as more desirable than other available alternatives. To test the basic hypothesis, we reduced the sample by this group of what might be termed *nonrational* respondents — people who could not substantiate their choice of facility in the manner in which we have prescribed. We reduced the sample by an additional seventy-two people who reported no use of any health facility during the preceding year.

To test the rationality of respondent answers, we compared *rational choice* and *actual choice*. We defined *rational choice* as the kind of facility (or facilities) that the calculation showed to have the greatest (or equally greatest) weightings. *Actual choice* was defined as the kind of facility (or facilities) that the person reported most (or equally most) utilized during the preceding year. In 80 precent of the cases, rational choice predicted actual choice. Of the forty respondents whose utilization we failed to predict, twenty-three were persons whose *closely-preferred choice* (wherein the calculation showed their second-most preferred weighting to be within 90 percent of their calculated rational choice) agreed with actual choice. If we make an allowance for the probable difficulty in the rank-ordering process that these people encountered and modify the previous definition of rational choice to include closely preferred choices, then the model predicted correctly 87 percent of the decisions.

We expected orginally that incorrect predictions would be most prevalent among low-income persons who might indicate a choice of private physician, but whose utilization would be greater of nonprivate sources. We thought that some people might be too embarrassed to acknowledge their actual lack of access to private physicians. As it turned out, while the predictions for those who used private sources were more accurate than for those who used nonprivate kinds of facilities, the overall prediction rates for all kinds of services were better among inner-city residents (91.5 percent) than among the remainder of the sample (86.5 percent). The model's weaker predictive power among users of different facilities in the non-inner-city portion of the sample appears to result from difficulty with the operationalization of the dependent variable actual choice.

In retrospect, some faults of the survey are apparent. For example, we did not control adequately for constraints on utilization associated with clinics at work. Presumably, some people whom we believed would prefer to use the clinic at work might have found this type of facility inaccessible on nights and weekends. Consequently, they may have reported greater use of a different facility. Similarly, some who might have preferred to use a private doctor may, because of company requirements, have had to use the clinic at work. We suspect also that some people may have found it difficult to distinguish their choice of facility solely on the basis of a presumed routine medical problem. As we later discuss, the factors that make an emergency room desirable as a source of emergency care are not necessarily the same factors that motivate a person to select a source for routine problems. We also know that some of the people who used the hospital clinic did so because they were referred to the hospital by their physician. Thus, while these people may have preferred to use a private physician, their actual choice emerged as the hospital clinic, because of factors that they could not control. Unfortunately we did not examine these now apparent possibilities. However, we did try to find out whether the individual's past medical utilization might have affected the model's predictive power. We wished to know, for example, whether those who made only one visit to any source were as predictable as those who reported larger numbers of visits. We found no significant change of predictive efficacy as frequency of utilization increased. Respondents appeared to act in rational conformity with their expectations even with minimal exposure to medical services.

In sum, the exercise appeared to validate the utility of the model of patient choice that we had created. Moreover, our assumptions about the rationality of human behavior also seemed to be justified. A relatively small percentage of people were unable to identify decision-components. Another small group found it difficult to rank-order components or to assess facilities. These totaled less than 10 percent of the sample. Thus the vast majority of the people demonstrated the characteristics of rational behavior that we had assumed. More importantly, between 80 and 86 percent of these actually manifested rational utilization of health-care facilities. In our view, these findings confirmed the reliability of the model and the validity of our use of the categories of decision-components as evaluative criteria.

The Choice of Emergency Care

We have suggested that the process of health-care utilization can be conceived as a sequential chain of decisions that culminates with the person's choice of a particular facility, and we have examined this decisional calculus in the context of care sought for the treatment of routine types of medical problems. Our intent was to derive the universe of criteria that people use to judge the utility of ambulatory-care sources. Consequently, for the purpose of evaluating the Genesee Health Service we were not concerned with how, why, or when the patient decided to seek care per se, only with how and why he chose a particular source. Nevertheless, the community survey did offer the opportunity to study some of the antecedent factors that prompt a person to want to seek care in the first place. We felt it important, for example, to attempt to find out why people use emergency rooms. Use of emergency-room facilities for nonurgent medical needs has increased. Genesee planners hoped that the new health service would tend to reduce this "inappropriate" use of Genesee's emergency facilities. We therefore incorporated in the survey protocol a set of questions on this subject.

Central and Volume Sources of Care

At the outset of the interview, respondents were asked to identify a primary and secondary *central* source of care, that which they felt they could always turn to when they needed medical help or advice. By definition, "the individual's central source of care is his focal medical source — not necessarily in point of time, sequence, or volume of use, but in its being to him the most important facility or physician to whom he turns when he needs medical care or advice."[8] We worded our opening question to reflect this definition. We used the respondent's reported utilization of care to calculate his *volume* source — that where he made the greatest number of visits. Table 2-5 presents our findings and shows that most people consider the emergency room as a substitute, rather than as a primary central source of care. From the data we also determined that more than half the sample had been to an emergency room at least once during their lives, and that 18 percent had been to one during the preceding twelve-month period. Only 1 percent of the sample reported more frequent use of the emergency room than any other source of care.

Table 2-5
Relationship between Central Source of Care and Volume Source of Care

Type Source	Primary[a] Central Source		Substitute[b] Central Source		Volume[c] Source	
	(%)	(No.)	(%)	(No.)	(%)	(No.)
Hospital emergency room	6	(27)	73	(318)	1	(4)
Hospital clinic	5	(22)	2	(9)	5	(24)
Private doctor	76	(332)	6	(27)	68	(296)
Clinic at work	2	(9)	1	(6)	5	(23)
Neighborhood health center	1	(6)	1	(6)	1	(5)
Multiple sources	—	—	—	—	3	(13)
None	9	(41)	16	(71)	17	(72)
Total	100	(437)	100	(437)	100	(437)

Source: William C. Stratmann and Ralph Ullman, "A Study of Community Attitudes About Health Care: The Role of the Emergency Room," *Medical Care* 13(1975):1033. With permission.

[a]"Is there any one place or person that you feel you can rely upon when you need help about a medical problem? Is there someone or some one place that you feel you can always turn to when you need medical help or advice?"

[b]"If for any reason this place were not available to you, to which of these (other) places would you go instead?"

[c]For routine problems.

Table 2-6
Relationship between Volume Source of Care and Use of Emergency Room

	Emergency Room Visit in Past Year			
	Yes		No	
Volume Source	*(%)*	*(No.)*	*(%)*	*(No.)*
Hospital emergency room	100	(4)	0	(0)
Hospital clinic	38	(9)	62	(15)
Private doctor	16	(46)	84	(250)
Clinic at work	17	(4)	83	(19)
Neighborhood health center	20	(1)	80	(4)
None (for routine problems)	14	(10)	86	(62)

Source: William C. Stratmann and Ralph Ullman, "A Study of Community Attitudes About Health Care: The Role of the Emergency Room," *Medical Care* 13(1975) :1033. With permission.

The likelihood of using an emergency room is about the same, regardless of the patient's volume source of care, with one notable exception. As table 2-6 indicates, people who are dependent primarily on the hospital clinic for routine care are twice as likely to use the emergency room as people who customarily use other sources of care. While it is clear that for most Rochester residents the emergency room is neither a primary central source of care nor a volume source of care, it is evident that local hospital emergency rooms are perceived by the local population to be important components of Rochester's health-care system.

Urgency of Medical Need

Interviewers documented the respondent's utilization of alternative types of medical facility and elicited the reasons for these reported visits, in particular, the urgency of the medical condition that prompted the respondent to seek care in the first place. In table 2-7 we show the reported urgency of the problems associated with the use of different types of medical facilities. Of the people who reported using an emergency room at one time or another, 95 percent stated that an urgent medical need prompted that visit. When we compare the central source of care of those people who have used an emergency room, with the perceived urgency of the problem that led to the visit (table 2-8), we find that 85 percent of the people who cite the emergency room as a central source of care assert their actual use of the emergency room to be associated with an urgent problem. For the group of people who cite the hospital outpatient clinic, the comparative figure is 93 percent, and, for those who use a private doctor, 97 percent.

Table 2-7
Reported Urgency of Problem That Prompted Use of Care Source

| | Urgency of Problem[a] | | | | | |
| | Urgent | | Nonurgent | | Total | |
Care Source	(%)	(No.)	(%)	(No.)	(%)	(No.)
Hospital emergency room	95	(213)	5	(11)	100	(224)
Hospital clinic	16	(16)	84	(82)	100	(98)
Private doctor "A"[b]	13	(53)	87	(341)	100	(394)
Private doctor "B"	18	(53)	82	(244)	100	(297)
Private doctor "C"	21	(30)	79	(115)	100	(245)
Clinic at work	40	(45)	60	(66)	100	(111)
Neighborhood health center	23	(5)	77	(17)	100	(22)

Source: William C. Stratmann and Ralph Ullman, "A Study of Community Attitudes About Health Care: The Role of the Emergency Room," *Medical Care* 13(1975):1033. With permission.

[a]"When you go to the (care source), is the problem so urgent that you have to see a doctor right away, or can you usually wait a while and put off seeing him until the next day?"

[b]Private doctor "A" is the most frequently used type of physician, "B" is the second most frequently used, "C" is the least frequently used.

Table 2-8
Urgency of Emergency Room Problem by Central Source

| | Urgency of Emergency Room Problem[a] | | | | | |
| | Urgent | | Nonurgent | | Total | |
Central Source	(%)	(No.)	(%)	(No.)	(%)	(No.)
Hospital emergency room	85	(17)	15	(3)	100	(20)
Hospital clinic	93	(14)	7	(1)	100	(15)
Private doctor	97	(155)	3	(5)	100	(160)
Clinic at work	100	(3)	0	(0)	100	(3)
Neighborhood health center	67	(2)	33	(1)	100	(3)

Source: William C. Stratmann and Ralph Ullman, "A Study of Community Attitudes About Health Care: The Role of the Emergency Room," *Medical Care* 13(1975) :1033. With permission.

[a]"When you go to a hospital emergency room, is the problem usually so urgent that you have to see a doctor right away, or can you usually wait a while and put off seeing him until the next day?"

It is apparent that the use of the emergency room is associated in the patient's mind with a symptom that he believes warrants immediate medical attention, a symptom that, to the patient, usually denotes an urgent medical problem. Yet, it is estimated that only about one-third of all emergency-room visits can be described objectively as urgent in nature. We must assume, therefore, that people tend to overestimate the severity of their

Table 2-9
Anticipated Availability of Physicians

A. Telephone Accessibility

"If you wanted to reach your (child's) doctor on the phone at night or on Sunday, how much trouble do you think you would have—a great deal, some, or no trouble at all?"

| | Medical Need | | | |
| | Adult | | Child | |
Anticipated Difficulty	(%)	(No.)	(%)	(No.)
Great deal	19	(71)	9	(23)
Some	29	(110)	29	(71)
No trouble at all	52	(197)	62	(151)
Totals	100	(378)	100	(245)

B. House Calls

"Suppose you were sick and wanted a (your child's) doctor to come to your house to examine you at night or on Sunday. How much trouble do you think you would have getting your doctor to come to your house—a great deal, some or no trouble at all?"

| | Medical Need | | | |
| | Adult | | Child | |
Anticipated Difficulty	(%)	(No.)	(%)	(No.)
Great deal	51	(192)	52	(116)
Some	25	(92)	24	(53)
No trouble at all	24	(90)	24	(52)
Totals	100	(374)	100	(221)

C. After-Hours Office Calls

"Suppose you simply wanted to see a doctor—not have him come to your home—and you were willing to go where he asked. How much trouble do you think you would have seeing your doctor at night or on Sunday—a great deal, some, or no trouble at all?"

| | Medical Need | | | |
| | Adult | | Child | |
Anticipated Difficulty	(%)	(No.)	(%)	(No.)
Great deal	16	(61)	13	(31)
Some	28	(106)	21	(53)
No trouble at all	57	(217)	66	(164)
Totals	101	(384)	100	(248)

(Table 2-9 continued)

D. Action in Event of Urgent Medical Need

"If you yourself (if one of your children) suddenly needed medical help at night or on a Sunday, what would you do?"

	Medical Need			
	Adult		Child	
Action Taken	(%)	(No.)	(%)	(No.)
Phone doctor	55	(237)	68	(177)
Call police or ambulance	5	(21)	2	(4)
Go to emergency room	35	(154)	26	(67)
Phone doctor and go to emergency room	2	(10)	3	(8)
Other	3	(13)	2	(4)
Totals	100	(435)	101	(260)

Source: William C. Stratmann and Ralph Ullman, "A Study of Community Attitudes About Health Care: The Role of the Emergency Room," *Medical Care* 13(1975):1033. With permission.

Note: In this table missing answers cause sample sizes to vary. Some tables do not sum to 100% because of rounding.

medical needs. But, however the problem is defined by either patient or provider, the patient's actions in selecting an appropriate source of care probably are influenced also by his perception of the accessibility of alternative sources. A Michigan Blue Cross study reports that many people before going to an emergency room first try unsuccessfully to locate their own physician.[9] Other people reportedly assume that their physician is not available. While our questionnaire unfortunately did not document whether the respondent had attempted to contact a physician before seeking help in the emergency room, of the 18 percent who used an emergency room in the last year, 70 percent reported also having used a private physician during that period. Thus many of the people who visited an emergency room were acquainted with a private physician. For one reason or another, they chose instead to go to an emergency room for care.

Physician Access

To examine the issue of physician accessibility, respondents were asked how they would go about getting help outside of normal office hours, for two different types of medical need. One set of questions dealt with adult needs for medical care; a second set concerned children's needs. These data are presented in table 2-9. Generally, it would seem that people believe their children's pediatrician to be more accessible than their own physician, although only about one-quarter of either group of physicians can be expected to make house calls. Many in the sample would proceed directly to an emergency room if they suddenly needed help at night or on Sunday.

Choosing an Emergency Room

Earlier we discuss at length the criteria that patients use to evaluate sources of ambulatory care for routine problems. We categorize these criteria as economic, temporal, convenience, sociopsychological, and quality factors. We now use these criteria to examine how people choose an emergency room, given an urgent medical need. Each respondent was asked, in the event he needed help for an urgent medical problem, which of several local emergency rooms he would go to and why. To enable a comparison of these responses with the reasons why people choose a source of care for routine problems, we aggregated for the emergency-room context the first reason cited by the respondent, and for the choice of a source for routine problems, the reason cited as most important by the respondent. These data are presented in table 2-10.

Table 2-10
Frequency of Mention of Most Important Decisional Criterion for Selection of Source of Care

	(1) Urgent Problem[a]		(2) Routine Problem[a]	
Most Important Criterion	(%)	(No.)	(%)	(No.)
Economic	–	(1)	2	(5)
Temporal	5	(12)	9	(22)
Convenience/location	79	(196)	14	(34)
Sociopsychological	2	(4)	7	(17)
Quality of care	14	(34)	68	(169)
Totals	100	(247)[b]	100	(247)[b]

Source: William C. Stratmann and Ralph Ullman, "A Study of Community Attitudes About Health Care: The Role of the Emergency Room," *Medical Care* 13(1975):1033. With permission.

[a]Column (1) represents criteria mentioned with respect to choice of an emergency room for urgent medical need. Column (2) represents criteria mentioned with respect to selection of care source for routine medical problems.

[b]The sample size is reduced by respondents who cited criteria that were either nonspecific or factors over which the respondent had no control, for example, reputation of facility or referral by another physician, and, therefore, do not enable categorization by the listed categories of utility criteria.

We determined that slightly more than half our sample cited location (a factor that we included in convenience criteria) as a major determinant in their selection of an emergency room from those available, given an urgent medical need. We also found that the vast majority of these people do, in fact, select the emergency-room facility closest to their homes. One might wonder, however, since an urgent condition should prompt people to hasten to the nearest emergency room for help, why more people did not mention location as the reason for their choice of emergency room. The explanation is simple. Hospitals in Rochester are clustered around the inner-city area, so that people living in the center of the city have nearly equal access to several emergency rooms. Logically, as the distance between alternative emergency rooms is reduced, we would expect people to trade off location for other things, perhaps quality of care or sociopsychological factors. When we divided our sample into inner-city and suburb subsamples in order to examine this hypothesis it became evident that location is relatively less important to the inner-city residents. Further, as table 2–11 shows, when the object of the patient's concern is a routine problem, and when we control for

Table 2-11
Relationship among Decisional Criterion, Location of Residence, and Type of Care Source

Most Important Criterion	(1) Choice of Emergency Room[a]				(2) Choice of Routine Care Source[a]			
	Suburb		Inner-City		Suburb		Inner-City	
	(%)	(No.)	(%)	(No.)	(%)	(No.)	(%)	(No.)
Economic	—	(1)	2	(1)	1	(5)	4	(5)
Temporal	4	(9)	13	(8)	7	(27)	9	(11)
Convenience	82	(205)	44	(27)	13	(47)	9	(10)
Sociopsychological	2	(4)	7	(4)	9	(31)	18	(21)
Quality of care	13	(32)	34	(21)	70	(254)	60	(71)
Totals	101[b]	(251)	100	(61)	100	(364)	100	(118)
	Chi-square $p < .01$				Chi-square $p < .01$			

Source: William C. Stratmann and Ralph Ullman, "A Study of Community Attitudes About Health Care: The Role of the Emergency Room," *Medical Care* 13 (1975): 1033. With permission.

[a]Column (1) represents criteria mentioned with respect to choice of an emergency room for urgent medical need. Column (2) represents criteria mentioned with respect to selection of care source for routine medical problems.

[b]Does not sum to 100% because of rounding.

the area in which the respondent lives, we observe a much smaller difference in the relative importance of a facility's location.

An Unanticipated Finding

The community survey questionnaire was demanding of respondents, and we were concerned about the extent to which a person's educational background might affect his understanding of the complex question format. We decided to pretest the questionnaire with some clinic patients, among whom we expected to find people with little formal education. To our surprise, the first randomly selected respondent reported that she had attended the Sorbonne, which prompted us to ponder briefly about the laws of probability. While this event is only of anecdotal interest, the survey itself yielded a more important unanticipated finding that we think worth mentioning.

A basic goal of Genesee's planners was good patient-provider rapport. Obviously personal communications were important to this goal. We decided to use the community survey to estimate the need for special language qualifications among GHS staff. In particular, we wanted to find out whether members of the Spanish-speaking community encountered language difficulties when they visited a hospital emergency room, which many used as a source of primary care. Thus, we asked all respondents whether they had ever experienced difficulty talking to the staff of a hospital emergency room because of language problems. We found that this was *not* a problem for Spanish-speaking patients, because they brought their own interpreter when they went to the emergency room. Our unexpected finding related to the *English-speaking* population, 10 percent of whom reported having experienced a language problem in the emergency room — with *foreign-speaking physicians.*

The Physician Survey

Although probably most important, the replacement of Genesee Hospital's outpatient clinics with a group medical practice was only one of several changes that were being made.[10] All ambulatory services were organized as a department with a full-time director, and substantial changes were anticipated in the emergency unit. While it was hoped that the new health service would lessen inappropriate emergency-room utilization, particularly among former clinic patients, Genesee's planners wanted to restructure the emergency services area so as to make it more functional and responsive to the obviously changing public demand for nonemergent services. To facilitate the planning process, we were requested to conduct a survey of physicians who used the hospital's emergency room, to solicit their views about how it might be improved. The need to conduct the survey presented an excellent opportunity to learn how physicians felt about standards that might be used to evaluate ambulatory-care services. Practical considerations dictated the use of a mailed survey questionnaire. We needed the widest possible input of ideas about proposed changes in the emergency room, but budgetary constraints precluded personal interviews with a large sample of physicians. While we harbored no illusions about being able to obtain the same richness of information that our community survey had yielded, we did hope to derive sufficient data to permit a general comparative analysis.

The need for opinion about how to improve the emergency room suggested that our primary population of respondents should consist of Genesee-affiliated physicians in all specialties. We also mailed the questionnaire to all other primary-care physicians in the area. A response rate of about one-third yielded a usable sample of 145 completed questionnaires, for the most part from Genesee-affiliated physicians. The portion of the questionnaire that solicited physician opinion about ambulatory care was divided into two sections. In one section the physicians were asked to define, in their own words, the criteria that they as professionals believed to be important as standards for the evaluation of ambulatory-care facilities. In a manner analogous to the community survey, they were asked to assign values of importance to these criteria. The universe of criteria were collapsed later into the five categories used in the consumer survey, and values were normalized to permit comparative analysis. Table 2–12 presents a summary of these data. Although the physicians assigned more weight than consumers to economic factors, this criterion again was least important. Time and sociopsychological factors were weighted approximately the same by

Table 2-12
Comparative Aggregated Relative Importance of Criteria for Physicians and Consumers

	Criterion[a]					N
	Economic	Temporal	Convenience	Sociopsychological	Quality	
	(%)	(%)	(%)	(%)	(%)	(%) No.
Physicians	7.3	9.4	11.8	20.2	51.3	100 (112)
Consumers	3.5	11.2	20.6	19.8	44.9	100 (521)

[a]Column percentages reflect the normalized weighted values of criterion importance for different row variables.

both groups. Curiously, the physicians weighted quality of care factors only slightly higher than did consumers. Of all criteria categories, the two samples differ most with respect to the relative importance of convenience factors, included in which are such things as accessibility, location, and continuity. Consumers clearly expressed greater concern about these factors than did the sample of physicians.

Another section of the questionnaire advised the physicians of a recent Rochester survey that had asked people to discuss how and why they chose a source of care for routine ambulatory-care problems. We described how the answers to that question had been categorized into five groups. With this introduction, we then asked the physicians to indicate, first, their own opinion of the relative importance of the criteria groups and, second, how they thought their patients might have evaluated the criteria. Table 2-13 presents these data. The sample of physicians apparently saw much similarity between their own opinion and that of their patients. They apparently also saw little difference in the manner in which male and female patients would interpret the importance of these criteria. This view is at odds with actual reported consumer opinion. The community survey showed that men

Table 2-13
Physician Views and Physician Opinion of Patient Views

Physician Opinion[a] of:	Criterion					
	Economic (%)	Temporal (%)	Convenience (%)	Sociopsychological (%)	Quality (%)	N (%) No.
Male patient views	19.4	17.5	18.8	20.5	23.8	100 (103)
Female patient views	17.7	19.9	19.5	19.6	23.4	100 (103)
Physician's own view	18.0	18.0	17.8	18.5	26.9	100 (103)

[a]The question read:
"We would like to find out now how you think your patients perceive the relative importance of these categories of evaluative factors.

If you are an obstetrician or a gynecologist please indicate how you think your adult patients would weight the categories of factors; if you are a pediatrician, how each parent would weight the factors; or, if you are in another type of practice, how your adult male and female patients would weight the factors.

Using the same scale as before, in the column below applicable to your specialty, write a number in the space(s) next to each category to indicate how you think your patients (or their parents) would weight the relative importance of the different categories of factors."

viewed convenience factors with much greater importance than did women, and sociopsychological factors with much less importance (see table 2–3). Thus, the data suggest a lack of appreciation by some physicians of patient expectations. It is evident from the community study that consumers do judge the overall process of care delivery. Notwithstanding the patient's awareness of his relatively passive role, he does manifest his displeasure at times. In the community survey, respondents also were asked if there was any source of care to which they would not return because of dissatisfaction with some aspect of the care they received. Almost one-third of the people who reported multiple use of a given type source of care responded in the affirmative. Their reasons were primarily related to excessive waiting time, poor interpersonal relations between themselves and the doctor or staff, and dissatisfaction with the medical treatment they received. Thus, while most physicians may be sensitive to patient feelings, some others apparently are not.

Summary

From our view, the study of utilization should begin at either one end or the other of the causal chain of decisions that represent this process, and one might argue for either strategy. The need to ascertain the standards by which people select their source of ambulatory care permitted us to test the theory of rational choice under circumstances that enable a simplified operationalization of the model constructs. Given the demonstrated viability of the model in this context, others may choose to apply it to the examination and explanation of antecedent decisions in the process of utilization, in particular to the study of the determinants of individual attitudes about health care.

Each ambulatory visit is the result of a consumer decision. Our objective was to understand the nature of that decision, and to describe the universe of decision-components that influence the consumer's choice of facility. We collapsed the decisional criteria into categories relating to the utility of cost, time, convenience, sociopsychological, and quality factors. We have discussed the relative importance of these criteria. It was not our intent to judge the wisdom of the consumer's perception of his biological or medical needs. Our study shows, however, that the consumer can explain his actions, that he does seem to know what he wants, and that his behavior is related to the purposeful pursuit of identifiable goals or values. One can argue that the average person is little qualified to judge the quality of medical care he receives. The decision to seek care, however, is an individual prerogative, and whether qualified or not people do evaluate the quality of care they receive, as well as other aspects of the process. However invalid consumer perceptions of the process of care may appear to the medical professional, patients' decisions do not appear to be either capricious or irrational, given the information to which they have access. The actions of our sample of respondents accord with their cognitive awareness of the relative utility of things that matter to them. Their decisions are rational, as we define this term.

Time, convenience, and interpersonal relations are of considerable importance to people, in many instances collectively more so than the quality of care. As we suggest, the explanation may be that to many people high levels of quality characterize all of their available alternative sources of care. As a consequence, the relevance of quality factors to the choice of facility is lower than one might expect. An apparent paradox is evident also with respect to the salience of economic criteria. We explain it in an analogous fashion. The high cost of medical care is a source of concern, both to consumers and to providers of care. Cost of care, however, does not seem to be a major factor in the patient's choice of facility. We assume that a consumer weighs the anticipated benefit of care for a perceived medical need against economic and temporal costs and the inconvenience of obtaining care, and that he decides to seek care only when he believes that the medical benefits will exceed the costs; but once he decides to seek care, the source of care he chooses is a function of factors other than cost. *Ceteris paribus*, patient satisfaction vis-à-vis these other decision-components would seem to be the *sine qua non* for the success or failure of any health service.

Our construct of the patient's decision process was intended to enable a determination of the identity and relative importance of the variety of factors that influence the use of health-care sources. Our results show also that people can and do distinguish between the attributes of emergency rooms, given an urgent medical need, just as they can distinguish between the attributes of other sources of care for routine problems. Many people express an overriding concern for the location of the emergency room, a matter that is prompted apparently by their perception both of the urgency of their medical problem and the accessibility of alternative health-care sources. Most people probably believe, logically, that the sooner a problem is treated the sooner their distress will be relieved. For some people, therefore, the discomfort or inconvenience caused by even a common cold is likely to prompt them to seek immediate medical relief from the most accessible professional source. If they do not expect their physician to be available, or if they are embarrassed to refer such a problem to their physician outside of office hours, or for similar reasons to impose on him during office hours, they may take their problem instead to the hospital emergency room where they know that anonymous professional help is available. Health-care utilization is a complex behavioral phenomenon. Many factors influence patient decisions, and, depending on the individual, with varying degrees of importance. It is within the province of the professional to appraise the urgency of a patient's medical needs, and admittedly most emergency-room problems by professional standards are not urgent. The fact is, however, from the patient's perspective, many of these problems appear to be urgent. To assert, as some do, that nonclinical matters should not be important, or to criticize patients because they do not conform to professional standards, is presumptuous.

The intuitive understanding that Genesee's planners had of patient expectations was to a great extent corroborated by our study of community attitudes about health care. The explanation of patient utilization is complex. The choice of facility obviously is not simply a consequence of one's sex, age, income, race, or whatever. Planners believed that people from all walks of life shared common health-related wants and desires. They planned the Genesee Health Service to appeal to a broad segment of the Rochester community. In a later chapter we examine the extent to which they succeeded in achieving this goal.

Notes

1. The concept of "central" source of care is discussed in Jerry A. Solon and Ruth D. Rigg, "Patterns of Medical Care among Users of Hospital Emergency Units," *Medical Care* 10 (1972):60.

2. The algorithm that we used to evaluate individual choice of source of care was first conceived to investigate the subject of electoral choice. See William C. Stratmann, "The Calculus of Rational Choice," *Public Choice* 17(1974):93. In that context the calculation is an expression of the expected utility of one candidate or another. Decision-components of electoral choice relate to political issues, personality of candidate, and so forth. If we substitute the term *facility* for *candidate*, we can calculate patient choice of care facility.

Expressed formally,

$$E(U_A) = \sum_{i=1}^{n} C_i F_i A$$

where:

$E(U_A)$	=	the weighted preference for facility A,
i	=	a given decision-component,
C	=	the *normalized* weighted value of a given decision-component,
F	=	the weighted satisfaction for a facility with respect to a specific decision-component, and
$F_i A$	=	the weighted satisfaction for facility A with respect to the ith decision-component.

3. In this regard see R. Duncan Luce and Howard Raiffa, *Games and Decisions* (New York: Wiley, 1957).

4. One can argue that a respondent's description of his likes and dislikes is simply a "rationalization" of his actions. This issue is discussed in Stratmann, "The Calculus of Rational Choice." In that study, which involved a three-man electoral contest, the model predicted the voter's second choice of candidate with considerable success. Additionally, that study examined the effect on predictive power of increasing numbers of decision-components. The data produced an asymptotic curve, in which efficacy increased from 67 percent (with the use of only one decision-component in the calculation) to 83 percent with five decision-components. No significant change in predictive efficacy was observed with the use of additional components. In the present study, therefore, we used in the algorithm only a respondent's first five decision-components. The electoral study yielded a predictive efficacy of 83 percent, which the use of closely preferred second choices increased to 91 percent. In view of the multiple choices involved and the plethora of components that respondents in that study identified, we conclude that few people are likely to be able to rationalize their choice with such apparent consistency. Because the application of the model of voting choice to the choice of health facility involved even greater methodological challenges, we did not believe it desirable to complicate the computational problem further by again examining the question of rationalization.

5. Public attitudes about health-care issues are a relatively unexplored subject. The issue of cost, although apparently not very important to the choice of a source of care, is of pervasive concern. For a discussion of this subject see William C. Stratmann et al., "A Study of Consumer Attitudes About Health Care: The Cost, Control, and Financing of Health Services," *Medical Care* 13(1975):659.

6. The Harris Survey, "The Harris Survey, September 13–22, 1973," Survey conducted for the United States Committee on Governmental Operations. Quoted in *Current Opinion*, 2 (February 1973):24.

7. Bruce Hillman and Evan Charney, "A Neighborhood Health Center: What the Patients Know and Think of Its Operation," *Medical Care* 10(1972):336.

8. Solon and Rigg, "Patterns of Medical Care."

9. Henry F. Vaughan, Jr., and Charles E. Gamester, "Why Patients Use Hospital Emergency Departments," *Hospitals* 40(1966):59.

10. Material in this section has been taken from William C. Stratmann, "Physician Perspectives of the Consumer's Choice of Ambulatory Care: A Comparative Analysis of Relevant Evaluative Criteria" (Paper delivered at the 76th Annual Meeting of the American Sociological Association, San Francisco, August 1975).

3 Ambulatory Utilization at Genesee

The community survey provided us with a mechanism for documenting broad patterns of care and for understanding the process of health-service selection and utilization. We desired to acquire detailed information about how that process had been reflected in the utilization of ambulatory services at Genesee. We also needed base-line data in order to measure the extent to which the Genesee Health Service attained the patient population and patterns of utilization that had been envisioned by its planners. Further, as we began to appreciate the methodological issues involved in constructing such a data base, we anticipated that the work might be a useful guide for the planning of similar programs at other hospitals.

The data to which we had access were those that hospitals customarily generate for operational reports — monthly and yearly counts of visits made to the various outpatient clinics and to the various service specialties of the emergency room. These statistics lend themselves to the comparison of Genesee with other community hospitals. The data shown in table 3-1 are from 1968, prior to any pertinent changes at Genesee. At that time, Genesee had 382 inpatient beds. In the same category (300–399 beds) were 291 voluntary community hospitals, which represented approximately 5 percent of all community hospitals in the United States. These hospitals provided about 12–13 percent of all inpatient and ambulatory services in the country. While almost all of these hospitals had emergency rooms, only about three-fourths had outpatient clinics.[1]

Table 3-1 demonstrates that total utilization of ambulatory services at Genesee was greater than would be expected for a voluntary hospital of its size. Note, however, that the distribution of visits between the clinics and the emergency room is disproportionate to other hospitals in the group. The total of 39,380 visits made to the Genesee emergency room in 1968 is much greater than average, while the total of 22,233 outpatient-clinic visits is well below average for those hospitals that provided the service.

The nation-wide perspective was reflected in utilization in the local area. Genesee's outpatient-clinic volume was dwarfed by that of Strong Memorial, the University of Rochester's teaching hospital, which is located only a few miles distant on the southern perimeter of the city. Genesee's emergency-room utilization was much greater, comparatively, about two-thirds that of Strong's. This was true also of several other hospitals in Rochester. During the 1960s and early 1970s, Genesee consistently treated

Table 3-1
A Nation-Wide Perspective, 1968

	Genesee Hospital	All Voluntary, 300–399-Bed Community Hospitals[a]
Provided an outpatient clinic?	Yes	74.2% did
Provided an emergency room?	Yes	97.6% did
Provided either ambulatory service?	Yes	98.6% did
Annual ambulatory visits	61,613	46,199[b]
Ambulatory visits per inpatient admission	4.3	3.8
Annual outpatient-clinic visits	22,233	38,800[b]
Annual emergency-room visits	39,380	17,200[b]
Outpatient-clinic visits as proportion of all ambulatory visits	36.1%	63.2%
Emergency-room visits as proportion of all ambulatory visits	63.9%	36.8%

[a] Data abstracted from Nora Piore, Deborah Lewis, and Jeannie Seeliger, *A Statistical Profile of Hospital Outpatient Services in the United States: Present Scope and Future Role* (New York: Association for the Aid of Crippled Children, 1971).

[b] Average among those hospitals that provided the service.

between one-fourth and one-fifth of all emergency-room visits in the city.[2] The annual rate of utilization increased substantially, from 22,000 visits in 1960, to about 39,000 visits in 1968, to approximately 46,500 visits in 1972. Meanwhile, clinic utilization increased only moderately, peaking at about 25,000 annual visits. The rapid increase in emergency-room visits received considerable attention from the hospital administration. As early as 1964, concern had been expressed about the "inappropriate" use to which the emergency room was being put. At that time, a study estimated that only one-third of the visits made to the Genesee emergency room did in fact require the immediate availability of hospital facilities.[3]

The comparisons and categorizations of visits afforded a summary view of utilization of ambulatory services at Genesee. We recognize that such data fill certain kinds of administrative needs. For example, categorization of arrivals by time of day and specialty of service is useful in determining an adequate schedule for staffing an emergency room. But broader planning of health services clearly should emphasize the *patient* as the object of that process. In this regard, the available information was lacking. We should note that this problem is pervasive and not related solely to hospital utilization data: "A major weakness in most health service statistics is their inability to count patients, in addition to visits and services, and to define and characterize the population group that generates these visits."[4]

In their customary form, hospital statistics are symptomatic of what often is portrayed as the traditional institutional approach to the delivery of ambulatory services. In most hospitals, the clinic or emergency room is readily accessible to whatever people come its way. Too often, however, these cases are received, treated, and then discharged as discrete units, with little or no attention paid to overall patterns of utilization and referral. Even those physicians and nurses who are motivated to provide the patient better management of his care are frustrated by clinic block scheduling, frequent rotation of housestaff, inadequate follow-up of broken appointments, and other organizational constraints. The institution simply does not distinguish between, say, one patient who makes several visits during a given period, and several patients, each of whom makes a single visit. The inability to make a similar distinction from the available statistics is consistent with the organizational orientation to "visits" as the units of output.

Clearly, we could not rely on visit statistics to provide us with an adequate understanding of patient utilization of hospital services for the period prior to the development of the Genesee Health Service. Such data are an inadequate informational resource for the planning of any hospital-based program that has an objective of changing the traditional approach to outpatient care. Our recognition of these factors led to the development of a profile of the *patient population* that generated the visits to Genesee's ambulatory facilities.

Methodological Issues

Given the absence of an enrolled population or a computerized data system, sampling methods are required in order to obtain information about utilization by a population of patients. When the research subject is hospital ambulatory services, however, where the most convenient samples are in the form of visits, important methodological issues arise.[5]

Visit samples usually can be drawn from sources such as logbooks, appointment sheets, billing forms, and laboratory slips. These samples readily can be used to identify the individuals who constitute a patient population, defined on the basis of the utilization of the subject service during a specified period. But the visit sample is not a representative selection of these patients. Since the probability of any patient's appearance in the sample is directly proportional to the number of visits made during the period studied, high-frequency users are likely to be overrepresented. Unless the sample data are weighted to adjust for this disproportionate selection, inferences about the size and characteristics of the patient population cannot be made. As we shall demonstrate, the adjustment process is quite simple, requiring only that each sampled visit be weighted by the inverse of the patient's visit frequency.[6]

The appropriate weight for each visit generally would be obtained from the medical record. That is, once a sample of desired size has been drawn from the universe of visits, the medical record of each identified patient is reviewed, and the number of visits made during the period under study is noted. At this time, all demographic and other patient characteristics of interest also can be obtained.

During the course of the coding process, several problems may arise. First, the coder may be tempted to discard a sampled visit if it duplicates a patient who has been sampled previously. Instead, however, such repetitions should be retained in the sample and treated as any other cases. To do otherwise would be to effect a consistent bias against a proportionate selection of visits made by patients having different utilization frequencies. This proportionate selection of visits is necessary if the weighting procedure is to yield an unbiased representation of patients. Although no differentiation should be made for *analytic* purposes as to whether a case is duplicated, it is useful to *identify* the patient repetitions so that each medical record need be reviewed only once.

The second problem that may occur in the coding process is difficulty in obtaining the patient medical record that corresponds to each sampled visit. An illegible name or incorrect medical unit number may be the source of the problem, or the record simply may be unavailable. As in any sampling procedure, bias results if missing cases in the sample are distributed differently than in the universe from which the sample is drawn. For example, if frequency of ambulatory utilization is correlated positively with frequency of impatient admission, then the unavailability of the records of recent inpatients would bias downward the estimate of the number of high-frequency users in the ambulatory population. If such a relationship is suspected, every effort should be made to obtain access to the missing records.

The third potential coding problem is a discrepancy between the visits listed within the sampling frame and those found within the medical records. This discrepancy, whether due to clerical errors or to known procedures, will lead to inaccurate results, since the weighting computation is formulated under the assumption that the two sources comprise precisely the same visits. The extent of this problem should be determined through preliminary sampling and investigation.

While the visit is probably the most important unit of service, more detail on the type of visit made and the care rendered may be desired. If so, the medical record would be expected to provide additional useful information on each sampled visit, and coding can proceed accordingly. Projection of these visit characteristics to the universe of visits of course does not require differential weighting. Often, however, it is useful to employ the patient's utilization frequency as a control in order to analyze more closely the demands for service that are placed on the facility by various patient groups.

Just as visits can be described more finely by the components of service rendered, so also can they be aggregated into a larger unit, or *episode*, that is, one or more visits that relate to the same medical condition.[7] In some outpatient specialty clinics, such as obstetrics and surgery, episodes and patients may correspond quite closely; in others, utilization by patients for multiple episodes of care would be common. While episodes cannot be sampled directly from the visit universe, they can be abstracted from the medical record. Analysis of episodes in relation to the total utilization of the facility is conducted then by treating their number and description as patient characteristics, which require weighting in the usual manner.

Study of a hospital's ambulatory-services patient population involves a documentation of use for multiple facilities—the emergency room and the various outpatient clinics—each of which generally provides its own sampling frame. But the use of services other than a particular sampled facility can be considered a patient characteristic, abstracted from the medical record, and analyzed accordingly. Thus, the extent to which the *same* patients have used a given combination of services can be investigated by employing a sample drawn from any of the facilities involved, provided that each case is weighted by the inverse of the number of visits made strictly to the sampled facility. For example, documenting emergency-room utilization by clinic patients can be initiated either by a sample drawn from emergency-room visits or by a sample drawn from clinic visits. Any difference in results should be attributable solely to sampling error.

Genesee Hospital employed the basic requisites for conducting research according to the design that has been outlined. A unit medical-record system covered all patient services.[8] Each visit to the emergency room was recorded on an encounter form, which was placed into the patient's folder at the conclusion of the visit. Outpatient-clinic visits were noted directly into a special section of the folder. In addition, emergency and outpatient personnel kept sequential logs of all visits made to their respective facilities. Preliminary examination indicated an almost complete correspondence between logged and recorded emergency-room visits. Somewhat less correspondence was indicated for certain of the outpatient clinics.

The twelve-month period July 1, 1971-June 30, 1972, just prior to any possible effects of the Genesee Health Service, was chosen for the utilization study. A period of this length was selected to facilitate comparison with other studies and to provide a reasonable representation of our concept of a patient population. By implication, then, at any point in time, a person is regarded as a user of the hospital's ambulatory services if at least one visit has been made in the previous twelve months.

A careful count revealed that the logs of the twelve-month period contained 46,527 emergency-room visits and 24,478 outpatient-clinic visits, exclusive of visits made by hospital employees and student nurses. A random sample of 750 visits then was selected from the emergency-room log, and random samples totaling 1,384 visits were drawn from the logs of the clinics. The latter sampling ratios were larger, so as to attain comparable precision in analyzing the utilization of individual clinics. In like manner, greater proportions (10 versus 5 percent) were drawn from the visit logs of the smaller outpatient subspecialities.

For the purpose of investigating patient utilization patterns, the twenty-four outpatient clinics were combined into nine major specialty groups, and the frequency of visits made to each group was determined. This permitted us to consider each clinic group as a separate facility and to examine utilization patterns among any combination of groups, as well as between a group and the emergency room. Table 3-2 presents the clinic group designations, sampling frames, and sample sizes employed in the study.

Medical records for each of the 750 cases in the emergency-room sample were found. For the clinic samples, 29 of the 1,384 cases either could not be matched with the proper medical record or were matched with a record unavailable at the time of the study. Each of these cases was replaced by the next visit listed on the clinic log. A check for repetition of patients in the samples did save substantial effort in the review of medical records. Seven emergency-room patients and 118 clinic patients were encountered twice. An additional twenty-six clinic patients were encountered three, four, or five times.

Information abstracted from the medical records permits analysis of three major categories of data. The first category comprises visit characteristics, which, other than identification of the specialty clinic to which a sampled outpatient visit was made, apply only to the emergency-room sample and include day and time of arrival, mode of arrival, type of complaint, services received, and disposition. The second category of data consists of patient characteristics, such as age, sex, race, residence, and source of payment. Lastly, documented utilization patterns include emergency-room visits, outpatient-clinic visits, hospitalizations, and hospital-days incurred at Genesee during the period of study.

The analysis developed in two major sections. First, we examined the utilization patterns of emergency-room patients and attempted to understand better the factors underlying the observed increases in volume. Second, we defined a patient population who appeared to depend on the hospital for primary care and who, therefore, constituted an important target group for the Genesee Health Service.

The Emergency-Room Population

Table 3-3 presents the complete distribution of the sampled emergency-room visits by the patient's frequency of utilization.[9] The data illustrate the

Table 3-2
The Utilization Sample

			Logged Visits[a] (Sample Size)	
Outpatient Clinics				
Dental			2,196	(110)
Eye			903	(45)
Gynecology			2,343	(117)
Maternity			2,374	(119)
Medical			3,819	(191)
Medical Specialties			2,664	(267)
Allergy	328	(33)		
Arthritic	81	(8)		
Cardiology	228	(23)		
Chest	167	(17)		
Dermatology	599	(60)		
Diabetic	559	(56)		
Endocrinology	151	(15)		
Gastrointestinal	51	(5)		
Hematology	128	(13)		
Neurology	124	(12)		
Oncology	51	(5)		
Psychiatry	39	(4)		
Renal	158	(16)		
Orthopedic			1,286	(64)
Pediatric			5,702	(285)
Surgical			3,191	(186)
Genito-urinary	393	(39)		
Podiatry	135	(14)		
Surgical	1,818	(91)		
Surgical Recall	845	(42)		
Total			24,478	(1384)
Emergency Room				
Total			46,527	(750)

[a]Hospital employee and student nurse visits excluded.

basic weighting technique used throughout the analysis. First, the sample distribution is projected to the universe of 46,527 visits. Then, the estimated number of patients in each visit-frequency group is derived by dividing the visit frequency into the estimated number of visits made by those patients. For example, on the basis of the visit sample, we estimate that 8,933 visits were made by patients each of whom made two visits during the year. Dividing the former figure by the latter yields about 4,467 — the estimated number of two-visit patients. Further, by controlling for the size of each visit-frequency group (or, equivalently, by weighting each sampled case by

Table 3-3
Emergency-Room Utilization Frequencies

Year's Emergency-Room Visits	Visit Sample	Proportion of Sample	Estimated Visits	Estimated Patients
1	439	58.5%	27,234	27,234
2	144	19.2	8,933	4,467
3	71	9.5	4,405	1,468
4	36	4.8	2,233	558
5	15	2.0	931	186
6	17	2.2	1,055	176
7	11	1.5	682	97
8	3	.4	186	23
9	5	.7	310	34
10	2	.3	124	12
11	3	.4	186	17
12	1	.1	62	5
20	1	.1	62	3
22	1	.1	62	3
34	1	.1	62	2
Totals	750	100%	46,527	34,286[a]

Source: Ralph Ullman, James A. Block, and William C. Stratmann, "An Emergency Room's Patients: Their Characteristics and Utilization of Hospital Services," *Medical Care* 13 (1975): 1011. Used with permission.
[a]Total is estimated directly and is not exact sum of column due to rounding of all entries.

Table 3-4
Emergency-Room Visit-Frequency Groups

Year's Emergency-Room Visits	Estimated Patients	Patients	Estimated Visits	Visits
1	27,234	79.4%	27,234	58.5%
2	4,467	13.0	8,933	19.2
3 +	2,586	7.5	10,360	22.3
Totals	34,286[a]	100%	46,527	100%

Source: Ralph Ullman, James A. Block, and William C. Stratmann, "An Emergency Room's Patients: Their Characteristics and Utilization of Hospital Services," *Medical Care* 13 (1975): 1011. Used with permission.
[a]Total is estimated directly and is not exact sum of column due to rounding of all entries.

the inverse of the visit frequency), we establish the correspondence between the sample and a correctly weighted sample of patients, each of whom made at least one visit during the twelve-month period.

The vast majority of emergency-room patients made infrequent use of the facility. From table 3-4, which is a condensed version of table 3-3, it is seen that the year's 46,527 visits were made by an estimated 34,286 different people (548 is the standard error of this estimate[10]). Only 7.5 percent of the total group, or an estimated 2,586 patients, visited the facility more than twice during the year. Their impact on the emergency room was substantial, however, comprising 10,360 visits, or 22.3 percent of all visits made to the facility.

Much of the following analysis is presented in a format designed to highlight the difference between the visit-frequency groups identified in table 3-4. This division of the patient population is arbitrary, but we believe that separating the one-visit patients from the three-or-more-visit patients affords a reasonable method of distinguishing between *infrequent* and *regular* emergency-room users, and it also retains categories of sufficient size for meaningful statistical analysis.

Patient Characteristics

As shown in table 3-5, males constituted more than half of the emergency-room patient population. Although females made slightly more visits per person than did males, the difference is not statistically significant. Nor is any relationship apparent between age and visit frequency. However, a striking difference with respect to race is seen. Although constituting only about one-quarter of all users, blacks represented almost half of all patients who made three or more visits. A strong association with visit frequency is established also for source of payment. Patients covered by Medicaid comprised about half of the high-frequency users, as compared to only 19 percent of the one-visit patients, most of whom were covered by Blue Cross or commercial insurance. Further analysis revealed that, of the two racial groups in the patient population, the association between source of payment and visit frequency held only for whites. For black patients, who were overrepresented generally among the regular users, Medicaid coverage did not increase significantly the likelihood of such utilization.

Our data show that the emergency room drew its patients from a wide area in Rochester and surrounding Monroe County. To describe better the relationship between residence and utilization, we defined three mutually exclusive areas:

1. *Hospital area*, with a wide mix of housing and socioeconomic population groups. In addition to Genesee, it also contained two smaller hospitals.
2. *Nearby inner-city area*, which included a high percentage of black and Medicaid-eligible residents. It contained no hospitals, although several, including Genesee, were reasonably accessible.
3. *Nearby suburbs*, with a predominantly white, middle- and upper-

Table 3-5
Selected Characteristics of Emergency-Room Patients

	Year's Emergency-Room Visits						Visits/
	1		*2*		*3 +*	*Patients*	*Visits*	*Patient*

	1		*2*		*3 +*		*Patients*	*Visits*	*Patient*
Sex									
Male	54.4%	(239)	47.9%	(69)	51.8%	(65)	53.4%	52.5%	1.3
Female	45.6	(200)	52.1	(75)	48.2	(60)	46.6	47.5	1.4
Totals	100%	(439)	100%	(144)	100%	(125)	100%	100%	1.4
N.S.[a]									
Age									
0-14	26.9%	(118)	31.9%	(46)	32.6%	(41)	28.0%	29.1%	1.4
15-64	62.9	(276)	58.3	(84)	61.7	(77)	62.2	61.9	1.3
65 +	10.3	(45)	9.7	(14)	5.7	(7)	9.8	9.1	1.3
Totals	100%	(439)	100%	(144)	100%	(125)	100%	100%	1.4
N.S.[a]									
Race									
White	78.9%	(343)	64.6%	(93)	55.1%	(69)	75.2%	70.8%	1.3
Black	21.1	(92)	35.4	(51)	44.9	(56)	24.8	29.2	1.6
Totals	100%	(435)	100%	(144)	100%	(125)	100%	100%	1.4
$p < .001$[a]									
Payment									
Medicaid	18.8%	(82)	39.6%	(57)	50.5%	(63)	23.9%	30.4%	1.7
Other third party	69.5	(303)	47.9	(69)	38.2	(48)	64.3	57.9	1.2
No third party	11.7	(51)	12.5	(18)	11.3	(14)	11.8	11.7	1.3
Totals	100%	(436)	100%	(144)	100%	(125)	100%	100%	1.4
$p < .001$[a]									

Source: Ralph Ullman, James A. Block, and William C. Stratmann, "An Emergency Room's Patients: Their Characteristics and Utilization of Hospital Services," *Medical Care* 13 (1975): 1011. Used with permission.

[a]N.S. = not significant. The chi-square distribution is used to test the sample for dependence between visit-frequency and the designated patient characteristic. Note that, since the distribution of the unweighted sampled *visits* does not necessarily reflect the *patient* distribution in a group covering more than one visit-frequency, an adjustment is made within the portion of the sample pertaining to the "3 +" group. Just as each sampled case is weighted by $1/i$ (where i is the visit-frequency) in a calculation pertaining to the patient population as a whole, so is each case within the "3 +" group weighted by $3/i$ to correct for the different probabilities of sampling patients within the group. The result is an estimate of the distribution obtained if all patients in the "3 +" group were sampled in the same proportion as were the three-visit patients. The process yields a total of 125 "cases" instead of the 167 visits actually sampled, and the resultant chi-square test is somewhat conservative.

income population. Residents were dependent on the city's hospitals for emergency services.

Using 1970 census figures, we computed rates of utilization for the three defined geographic areas. Table 3-6 shows that, of the population who resided proximate to the hospital, an estimated 15.7 percent visited the

Table 3-6
Estimated Emergency-Room Utilization Rates for Selected Geographic Areas

	Hospital Area	A Nearby Inner-City Area	Nearby Suburbs
Patients	7,078	2,507	5,732
Visits	10,086	4,414	6,735
Population (1970)	44,980	22,218	132,536
Patients/1,000	157	113	43
Visits/1,000	224	199	51
Visits/patient	1.4	1.8	1.2

Source: Ralph Ullman, James A. Block, and William C. Stratmann, "An Emergency Room's Patients: Their Characteristics and Utilization of Hospital Services," *Medical Care* 13 (1975): 1011. Used with permission.

emergency room at least once during the year, a rate considerably higher than for either of the other areas. By contrast, the unweighted visit rates for the hospital and inner-city areas are not substantially different, because of the higher visits-per-patient frequency of the latter. We conclude that, because of socioeconomic factors, the inner-city resident was the most likely to use an emergency room as a regular source of care but chose that source from among several equally accessible facilities. The hospital-area residents had a clearer choice for the relatively fewer occasions when an emergency room was used. We should note that we would have been unable to analyze these relationships if the unweighted visit sample had been the only source of information.

Visit Characteristics

We had hypothesized various associations between visit arrival patterns and frequency of visit. In particular, a presumption that high-frequency users came more often at their "convenience" had led us to expect differences in the distributions of arrivals by time of day, and by weekday versus weekend. However, a categorization of all sampled arrivals into three eight-hour periods (12 A.M.–8 A.M.: 14 percent; 8 A.M.–4 P.M.: 45 percent; 4 P.M.–12 A.M.: 41 percent) is similar to that observed for each of the three visit-frequency groups. Further, a generally uniform distribution of visits by day of week does not differ significantly among frequency groups. Lastly, the likelihood of a visit arriving by ambulance was 10–12 percent, regardless of the number of visits made by the patient during the year.

Table 3–7 presents the visit characteristics for which significant associations with utilization frequency were found. First, a categorization by type of complaint reveals that visits made by high-frequency users were less likely to have been prompted by an accidental injury than were visits made by one-visit patients. Second, visits made by the latter group were more likely than the former to receive services (mostly laboratory tests, x-rays, and sutures) additional to examination by a physician. Further analysis revealed that this relationship held irrespective of type of complaint. Third, the patient's visit frequency is associated positively with a disposition through referral to an outpatient clinic and negatively with referral to a private physician. These last trends are not surprising, given our knowledge of the effects of residence, source of payment, and the visit frequency itself. All convey a dependence of the high-frequency emergency-room user on the hospital for ambulatory services. What is surprising is the small difference in rates of admission to the hospital. Despite making at least three times as

Table 3-7
Selected Characteristics of Emergency-Room Visits

| | Year's Emergency-Room Visits | | | | | | |
	1		2		3 +		Visits	
Type of Complaint								
Accident	48.5%	(213)	37.5%	(54)	23.4%	(39)	40.8%	(306)
Nonaccident	51.5	(226)	62.5	(90)	76.6	(128)	59.2	(444)
Totals	100%	(439)	100%	(144)	100%	(167)	100%	(750)
$p < .001$								
Services Received								
None/exam only	30.8%	(135)	34.0%	(49)	46.1%	(77)	34.8%	(261)
Additional services	56.0	(246)	56.3	(81)	42.5	(71)	53.1	(398)
Admitted	13.2	(58)	9.7	(14)	11.4	(19)	12.1	(91)
Totals	100%	(439)	100%	(144)	100%	(167)	100%	(750)
$p < .01$								
Disposition								
None/home	48.3%	(212)	43.8%	(63)	41.3%	(69)	45.9%	(344)
Private MD	21.9	(96)	20.8	(30)	13.8	(23)	19.9	(149)
OPD	12.1	(53)	22.2	(32)	25.7	(43)	17.1	(128)
Admitted	13.2	(58)	9.7	(14)	11.4	(19)	12.1	(91)
Other	4.6	(20)	3.5	(5)	7.8	(13)	5.1	(38)
Totals	100%	(439)	100%	(144)	100%	(167)	100%	(750)
$p < .001$								

Source: Ralph Ullman, James A. Block, and William C. Stratmann, "An Emergency Room's Patients: Their Characteristics and Utilization of Hospital Services," *Medical Care* 13 (1975): 1011. Used with permission.

Note: The chi-square distribution is used to test the sample for dependence between visit-frequency and the designated patient characteristic. In this case, no weighting procedure is necessary, since the distribution of the sampled visits is precisely the object of the analysis.

many visits, on any given visit the high-frequency user was almost as likely to be admitted to the hospital as was the one-visit patient.

Clinic and Inpatient Utilization

The categorization of visit dispositions provides an indication of the relationship between the emergency-room patient and utilization of the hospital's outpatient clinics. Clinic referrals did not necessarily result in kept appointments, however, nor were they the only means of generating clinic visits. Table 3–8 gives a broader perspective of this issue by identifying the proportions of emergency-room patients who made at least one outpatient-clinic visit during the study period. As shown, a strong positive association existed between frequency of visits to the emergency room and outpatient utilization. The weighted calculations yield an estimate of 4,804 as the number of patients who used both facilities. These patients made an estimated 10,360 visits to the emergency room and 13,893 visits to the outpatient clinics, or 24,253 total ambulatory visits, an average of 5 visits per patient. They generated about 57 percent of the year's outpatient volume.

The proportion of emergency-room patients who were admitted to the hospital as inpatients during the year is presented also in table 3–8. Consistent with the rather even disposition rates of emergency-room visits, a positive relationship exists between the emergency-room-visit *frequency* and

Table 3-8
Utilization of Other Services by Emergency-Room Patients

	Year's Emergency-Room Visits						
	1		*2*		*3 +*		*Patients*
Year's OPD Visits							
None	92.5%	(406)	66.0%	(95)	52.2%	(65)	86.0%
One or more	7.5	(33)	34.0	(49)	47.8	(60)	14.0
Totals	100%	(439)	100%	(144)	100%	(125)	100%
$p < .001$[a]							
Year's Inpatient Admissions							
None	82.9%	(364)	76.4%	(110)	70.0%	(88)	81.1%
One or more	17.1	(75)	23.6	(34)	30.0	(37)	18.9
Totals	100%	(439)	100%	(144)	100%	(125)	100%
$p < .01$[a]							

Source: Ralph Ullman, James A. Block, and William C. Stratmann, "An Emergency Room's Patients: Their Characteristics and Utilization of Hospital Services," *Medical Care* 13 (1975): 1011. Used with permission.

[a]See footnote to Table 3-5.

the likelihood of hospitalization. An estimated 30 percent of the high-frequency users were admitted to the hospital at least once during the year, as contrasted to only 17 percent of the one-time patients.

While the direct admission of emergency-room visits is recognized generally as an important source of inpatient "business,"[11] the overlap of inpatients and emergency-room patients during a given year provides further evidence of the strong interrelationship between the two services. Table 3-9 shows that about one-third of the admissions experienced by Genesee emergency-room patients in fact were not related directly to the disposition of an emergency-room visit. The estimated 8,266 total admissions of the population represent about 53 percent of all admissions to Genesee during the year. Due to the relatively long lengths of stay associated with these admissions, the effect on inpatient days was even more pronounced. An estimated 68 percent of the hospital's total inpatient-days were consumed by the emergency-room patient population.

The Primary-Care Patient Population

The term *primary care* has numerous connotations. For our purposes, the primary-care population consisted of patients who appeared to have utilized Genesee as a regular source of ambulatory care and whose required care seemed appropriate for management by the physicians of the Genesee Health Service.[12] We defined the *current* primary-care population as all patients who had made at least one visit to either the pediatric, gynecology, maternity, general medical, or medical subspecialty clinics during the year of the study. By defining the patient population in terms of the outpatient structure the analysis was simplified greatly, although in doing so the precision obtainable from a more detailed review was sacrificed.

Table 3-9
Estimated Inpatient Utilization by Emergency-Room Patients

| | Emergency-Room Visits | | | |
	1	*2*	*3+*	*All*
Emergency-room visits admitted	3,598	868	1,179	5,645
Other admissions	1,923	528	170	2,621
Total admissions	5,521	1,396	1,349	8,266
per patient	.20	.31	.52	.24
Average stay (days)	9.9	7.7	9.7	9.5
Total inpatient days	54,592	10,794	13,071	78,457
per patient	2.0	2.4	5.1	2.3

Source: Ralph Ullman, James A. Block, and William C. Stratmann, "An Emergency Room's Patients: Their Characteristics and Utilization of Hospital Services," *Medical Care* 13 (1975): 1011. Used with permission.

Medical subspecialty patients were included in the primary-care population because the great majority of them were dependent on the hospital for ambulatory services and presumably would benefit from the medical supervision afforded by a primary-care program. We perceived that many patients patronized the subspecialty clinics simply because there was no primary-care physician in the outpatient area (or elsewhere) to whom they could turn for the management of their more general problems. The same argument could be made for some of the frequent users of the emergency room. For several reasons, however, we decided to exclude the emergency-room visits from the primary-care sampling frame:

1. The number of frequent users was relatively small compared to the overall emergency-room population.
2. Of the high-frequency users, approximately one-third also made at least one visit to a primary-care clinic and therefore were included already in the defined population. Of the remainder, some made visits only for accidents or "true" emergencies, which we did not consider to be in the category of primary care.
3. The emergency-room staff made it a practice to identify patients who had no private physician and to refer them to the outpatient clinics for follow-up care. Those patients who chose not to accept these referrals may have been expressing a preference for their current pattern of utilization, which made it problematic whether they would accept referral to the new program.

Table 3-10 presents the primary-care population, which we estimated by applying the weighting technique to the visit samples from the designated clinics. The division of the population into pediatrics, medicine, and obstetrics/gynecology corresponds to the major specialties of the Genesee Health Service. The figures in parentheses indicate the numbers of patients estimated to have used more than one clinic group. As shown, the total primary-care population comprises approximately 6,000 patients. If we were to add some of the emergency room's frequent users not included already, the size of the primary-care population would increase somewhat, perhaps to about 7,000 patients.

Table 3-11 summarizes the utilization patterns, both ambulatory and inpatient, of the primary-care patients. For the present purposes, probably the major finding is the high rate of emergency-room utilization apparent for all three groups in the population. We think it reasonable to infer that, for many of these patients, the hospital, and not the clinic per se, was envisioned as the source of care.

In chapter 4 we discuss the growth and utilization of the new health service, using as a base for comparison the former primary-care population. To avoid redundancy, we omit here a documentation of the clinic population's sociodemographic characteristics and note only the following findings:

Table 3-10
Estimated Primary-Care Patient Population

Specialty Clinic		Patients
Pediatrics		2,563
Medicine		2,128
General medical	1,582	
Subspecialties	756	
(Less: both)	(210)	
Ob/Gyn		1,538
Gynecology	1,323	
Maternity	581	
(Less: both)	(366)	
(Less: pediatrics and medicine)		(25)
(Less: pediatrics and ob/gyn)		(15)
(Less: medicine and ob/gyn)		(299)
Total		5,890

Source: Ralph Ullman et al., "Study Provides Data for Planning Hospital-Based Primary Care," *Hospitals, J.A.H.A.* vol. 49, no. 22 (November 16, 1975): 75. Used with permission.

Table 3-11
Estimated Utilization of Hospital Services by the Primary-Care Patient Population

	Pediatrics	Medicine	Ob/Gyn	All
Patients	2,563	2,128	1,538	5,890[a]
Clinic visits within specialty	5,702	6,483	4,717	16,902
Per patient	2.2	3.0	3.1	2.9
Other primary-care-clinic visits	71	1,015	1,002	—
Per patient	0.0	0.5	0.7	—
Percent at least one visit	2%	15%	20%	—
Dental, eye, and surgical visits	509	1,490	1,098	2,774[a]
Per patient	0.2	0.7	0.7	0.5
Percent at least one visit	9%	27%	19%	17%
Emergency-room visits	3,009	3,416	2,305	7,856[a]
Per patient	1.2	1.6	1.5	1.3
Percent at least one visit	57%	65%	56%	59%
Inpatient admissions	192	536	663[b]	1,193[a]
Per patient	0.1	0.3	0.4	0.2
Percent at least one admission	7%	22%	38%	18%
Average stay (days) per admission	7.2	10.2	5.2	7.6
Total inpatient days	1,389	5,484	3,454	9,015[a]

Source: Ralph Ullman et al., "Study Provides Data for Planning Hospital-Based Primary Care," *Hospitals, J.A.H.A.* vol. 49, no. 22 (November 16, 1975): 75. Used with permission.
[a]Not the sum of the specialties, because of multiple use.
[b]Includes 350 obstetric admissions.

1. The age distribution of the existing primary-care population suggested that pediatric care for newborns and maternity care for teenagers would require emphasis in the new program.

2. The concept of a geographic "target" area, such as customarily associated with a neighborhood health center, did not fit Genesee's primary-care population. Patients came to Genesee from throughout the city. Only one-fifth of the approximately 6,000 patients came from the 45,000 residents of the hospital area.

3. About 65 percent of the primary-care patients had Medicaid coverage. Given the existing cost reimbursement policies of New York State, this distribution of patients was viewed by planners as favorable to the financial stability of the new program. However, the estimated 12 percent of the population for whom no third-party reimbursement source could be identified did present a clear financial risk to the program.

Discussion

It has been suggested that, to varying degrees in any institution, the emergency room plays three major roles: a trauma treatment center, a physician substitute when one's customary source is not available, and a family "physician" to the urban poor.[13] The community survey had demonstrated the widespread disposition of consumers to utilize emergency rooms in the second of these roles. Yet, we frankly were surprised that the Genesee-based sample of *users* displayed much the same pattern of behavior. Notwithstanding the urban location and the large volume of nonemergent problems, it is apparent that only a small proportion of the patient population considered the emergency room as their regular source of care. Rather, the majority of patients, who were generally white, insured, and from areas other than the inner city, utilized the facility only infrequently. The same behavioral phenomenon has been observed elsewhere. It is apparent that, for most of its patients, the emergency room "occupies a peripheral place in their system of care."[14]

The dominance of the infrequent user should not obscure the substantial number of patients who made multiple emergency-room visits during the year and whose consequent demands on the facility were considerable. These patients disproportionately were black, low-income, inner-city residents, who often also used the hospital's outpatient clinics. They had limited access to private physicians and apparently depended on the hospital as a regular source of ambulatory care, a pattern long recognized by other studies.[15],[16]

Three-fourths of the visits made by the emergency room's high-frequency users were for reasons other than accidental injury. About half apparently involved nothing more in the way of services than the attention of a physician. Nevertheless, we do not interpret this utilization as frivolous or unwarranted. On the contrary, the finding that 30 percent of these patients also incurred one or more hospital admissions during the period of the study shows that their health problems generally were serious enough to merit considerable attention.

Given the demonstrated overlap between the emergency-room and outpatient-clinic populations, it was not surprising to find high rates of emergency-room utilization for the more narrowly defined primary-care population. While the latter data did indicate an opportunity for the Genesee Health Service to reduce substantially the amount of emergency-room utilization by these patients, the total number of their visits was nevertheless rather small in comparison to the overall volume of 46,527 visits. Consequently, our expectations as to the immediately observable effect of the new program on the emergency room were diminished.

Placing the results of the study with those of the community survey and the known longitudinal trends of visit volume, we must conclude that the increase in ambulatory utilization at Genesee is only partly attributable to a relocation of private physicians from the inner-city area. A more important factor appears to be an increased use of the emergency room by a population to whom physicians were still generally available, but less accessible because of changing patterns of private practice. Thus, although the hospital is located in reasonable proximity to the inner city, its longitudinal pattern of ambulatory-care utilization prior to development of the Genesee Health Service appears more characteristic of a suburban institution.[17]

We realized that our assessment of the new program had to be done within the context of the results presented in this chapter. The rather small size of the population who depended on the hospital for primary health care seemed particularly important to this assessment, and we believed that the administrative task of transferring these patients to a new mode of care had to be evaluated accordingly. Similarly, we knew that the ability of the Genesee Health Service to attain its various objectives would be influenced by the existing pattern of ambulatory-care utilization at the hospital.

Notes

1. All comparative data are from Nora Piore, Deborah Lewis, and Jeannie Seeliger, *A Statistical Profile of Hospital Outpatient Services in the United States: Present Scope and Future Role* (New York: Association for the Aid of Crippled Children, 1971).

2. Richard Wersinger, *Emergency Department Utilization in Monroe Country, New York* (Rochester, N.Y.: Genesee Region Health Planning Coucil, 1971).

3. David N. Kluge, Robert L. Wegryn, and Bernice R. Lemley, "The Expanding Emergency Department," *Journal of the American Medical Association* 191(1965):801.

4. Jane H. Murnaghan, "Review of the Conference Proceedings," in *Ambulatory Care Data: Report of the Conference on Ambulatory Medical Care Records*, edited by Jane H. Murnaghan (Philadelphia: J. B. Lippincott Co., 1973), p. 17.

5. Portions of the material in this section have been presented as Ralph Ullman and William C. Stratmann, "Developing a Profile of Ambulatory Utilization" (Paper delivered at the 101st Annual Meeting of the American Public Health Association, San Francisco, November 4-8, 1973); Ralph Ullman, "Developing a Profile of Ambulatory Utilization: A Sampling Technique," in *Proceedings of the Public Health Conference on Records and Statistics: 15th National Meeting*, DHEW Publication No. (HRA) 75-1214 (Rockville, Md.: U.S. Department of Health, Education, and Welfare, 1975), pp. 207–210; and Ralph Ullman, "The 'Patient' and the 'Visit': A Basic Distinction in Health Services Research," mimeographed (Philadelphia: National Health Care Management Center, University of Pennsylvania, 1979).

6. The first application of this weighting procedure to health-services utilization appears to be Raymond C. Lerner and Corinne Kirchner, "Social and Economic Characteristics of Municipal Hospital Outpatients," *American Journal of Public Health* 59(1969):29. That application, however, calculates each weight from the number of visits made in the twelve months prior to the sampled visit rather than from the number of visits made within a fixed twelve-month period, as in the present study. More recently, the method recommended here has been formalized to study the characteristics of hypertensive patients treated in the medical clinic of a teaching hospital. See Donald S. Shepard and Raymond Neutra, "A Pitfall in Sampling Medical Visits," *American Journal of Public Health* 67(1977) :743. Additional comments related to the various approaches are found in Donald S. Shepard and Raymond Neutra, "Addendum to Article on 'Visit-Based Sampling,'" letter to the editor, *American Journal of Public Health* 69(1979) :954. Ullman, "The 'Patient' and the 'Visit'" presents a comprehensive literature review and discussion.

7. Jerry A. Solon et al., "Delineating Episodes of Medical Care," *American Journal of Public Health* 57(1967) :401.

8. Survey results indicate that only 67 percent of all hospitals that had an organized outpatient department employed such a unit medical record system covering at least the outpatient visits. From James P. Cooney, "The Community Hospital: Ambulatory Services, Statistics, and Medical Care Record Data," (Paper delivered at the Conference on Ambulatory Medical Care Records, Chicago, April 18-22, 1972).

9. This section is adapted from an article that appeared previously as Ralph Ullman, James A. Block, and William C. Stratmann, "An Emergency Room's Patients: Their Characteristics and Utilization of Hospital Services," *Medical Care* 13(1975):1011. Used with permission.

10. As calculated from equation (3) in Shepard and Neutra, "A Pitfall in Sampling Medical Visits."

11. John D. Thompson and Samuel B. Webb, Jr., "Effect of the Emergency Department on Hospital Inpatient Services: A Statewide Analysis," *Inquiry* vol. 10, no. 2 (June 1973):19.

12. This section is adapted from an article that appeared previously as Ralph Ullman et al., "Study Provides Data for Planning Hospital-Based Primary Care," *Hospitals, J.A.H.A.* vol. 49, no. 22 (November 16, 1975):75.

13. Paul R. Torrens and Donna G. Yedvab, "Variations among Emergency Room Populations: A Comparison of Four Hospitals in New York City," *Medical Care* 8(1970):60.

14. Jerry A. Solon and Ruth D. Rigg, "Patterns of Medical Care among Users of Hospital Emergency Units," *Medical Care* 10(1972) :60.

15. Joel J. Alpert et al., "The Types of Families that Use an Emergency Clinic," *Medical Care* 7(1969) :55.

16. E. Richard Weinerman et al., "Yale Studies in Ambulatory Medical Care: V. Determinants of Use of Hospital Emergency Services," *American Journal of Public Health* 56(1966):1037.

17. Stephen M. Davidson, "Understanding the Growth of Emergency Department Utilization," *Medical Care* 16(1978):122.

4

From Outpatient Clinic to Group Practice

In July 1971, simultaneously with the receipt by Neighborhood Health Centers of Monroe County, Inc. of the grant from the Office of Economic Opportunity, a Department of Ambulatory Services was created at Genesee Hospital. The outpatient clinics became the Outpatient Division (OPD), and the emergency room became the Emergency Division (ED). With the new Genesee Health Service (GHS), these two divisions thus were unified administratively under the leadership of a single director, a pediatrician who had been a consultant to NHC during the planning of the network and instrumental in the creation of the program at the hospital. Plans for the development of GHS and the phased termination of OPD were begun immediately.

At the time the research unit was started in July 1972, construction of the new GHS facility was well under way. The health service was to occupy the entire lower floor of the hospital's adjacent doctors' office building. Administrative offices for the Department of Ambulatory Services were located in the same building. In these spaces, which also contained two small treatment rooms, the director of the department and the newly appointed GHS Medical Director, also a pediatrician, had begun seeing patients in January 1972. When two additional pediatricians were hired in July, the transfer of patients from the pediatric and well-baby clinics was initiated. Also recruited was the first GHS internist, who continued to practice in his existing private office near the hospital but accepted referrals from OPD. All of these separate practices were moved into the main facility when it was opened in March 1973.

During the period of transition that accompanied the construction of the new facility, the OPD's pediatric, medical, and ob/gyn clinics were closed one by one, as additional GHS physicians were recruited. Most of the patients of these clinics were referred directly to GHS. Only a small proportion required referral to subspecialists for further care.

A variety of arrangements were made for OPD clinics that did not fit the primary-care model of GHS. The dental clinic had been subsumed already by the hospital's Department of Dentistry, which was housed in a newly constructed facility. The genito-urinary clinic, while technically considered a part of OPD, had been administered independently and conducted within the hospital's inpatient area. Its operation continued in that fashion. The ENT, eye, and podiatry clinics were terminated, with arrangements made for outside practitioners to see patients on referral from GHS or the hospital. The orthopedic and surgical clinics, which primarily treated emergency-room referrals, were moved to another location in the hospital and eventually came under the auspices of the Emergency Division. Sessions of the surgical postoperative clinic were scheduled in the new GHS facility, with physicians provided through the hospital's residency program. The physical space made available by the closing of OPD later was renovated and transformed into a community mental-health center.

As researchers, we faced several conflicting goals during the hectic period of construction and organizational change. We were anxious to formulate the overall research strategy and, subsequently, to begin designing the community survey and the ambulatory utilization study. But we also realized that any opportunity to examine the base-line facility, the OPD, would soon be lost. Already the pediatric clinic had changed greatly, and the pattern was to be repeated for other clinics. Compelled to compromise, we decided to invest a modest amount of time in examining some of the more frequently cited characteristics of care delivered in the hospital clinic setting. While the undesirable physical attributes of the clinics were readily apparent, we maintained a natural skepticism toward other criticisms commonly directed at such facilities.[1]

The Outpatient Clinics

For many years Genesee Hospital had operated a collection of specialty clinics, known informally as the Outpatient Department and scheduled for specific periods during weekdays. The term OPD customarily was used also in reference to the first-floor facility in which most of the clinic sessions were held. The most prominent feature of this facility was its large rectangular waiting area, on two sides of which one could enter a series of connected treatment rooms. A nurses' station was located in the middle of the area, and in one corner was a business office and cashier's window. At the cashier's window there stood, perhaps symbolically, a foot-high, tree-like metal structure holding a large number of rubber stamps, some of which we suspected had not been used for years.

We think it fair to characterize the facility as unattractive. The walls were of tile designed for function rather than appearance. While the molded-plastic chairs arranged throughout the waiting room seemed adequate, we were informed that the "hard benches" of tradition had been replaced only after formation of the Department of Ambulatory Services. Most importantly, however, provision for the privacy of patients was lacking. Preliminary tests such as weighing and blood pressure were done through open doors in view of the waiting areas, and patients who were asked to provide urine samples had to carry their specimens through the waiting room.

The scheduling of individual clinics was negotiated with the respective departments and reflected the number of patients who sought treatment. Major clinics, such as maternity and general medical, were scheduled four times a week, while small subspecialty clinics such as hematology might be held only once every two weeks. Often, two or more clinics would be conducted simultaneously. Visits were scheduled by appointment, although frequently in a *block* format that required all patients to arrive at the same time for a particular clinic session.

Physician staffing for the clinics was furnished through the hospital's medical education program and by the medical staff, who usually served on a voluntary basis. Arrangements varied greatly from one clinic to another. Nursing support was the responsibility of a core of registered nurses, who also performed many administrative functions and, in effect, "ran" the operation.

A bookkeeper and secretarial staff handled most OPD billing. Generally, a fee ($8.00 in the most recent years) was charged for the clinic visit itself, with additional charges for ancillary services (mainly x-ray, laboratory, and pharmacy) also billed by OPD. Collection procedures were lax. No follow-up billing existed, and a patient's payment record was seldom, if ever, cause for the denial of service. The Outpatient Department was recognized as a source of "charity" care for individuals who could not afford a private physician, and its financial structure reflected this tradition.

OPD "financing" changed considerably on implementation of the Medicaid program, for which the majority of clinic patients qualified. Under New York State rulings, for each Medicaid visit the hospital was reimbursed a flat rate according to the average total cost of the visit, including ancillary services. The rate, which was subject to approval by state authorities, was computed by the hospital's financial staff based on expenses incurred directly by OPD, such as nursing salaries, and on allocations of indirect expenses, such as plant maintenance and medical education.

Patterns of Operation

The processing and scheduling of OPD patients was the focus of a study that we conducted over a two-week period while all of the clinics except pediatric still were functioning at near normal levels.[2] The nursing and clerical staffs assisted in recording each patient's time of arrival at OPD and times of entrance to and exit from the examination rooms. Routinely collected data sources, such as appointment lists and daily census sheets, were obtained and checked for accuracy. A total of 672 visits were recorded during the period of study.

The data indicated that an appointment system was enforced in OPD. Only 10 percent of all visits were walk-ins—visits made without an appointment. However, patients frequently failed to keep their appointments. Although the no-show rates were high—39 percent over all clinics—we observed that OPD was not handicapped seriously, because of its block appointment system and first-come, first-served policy. Once all patients had been seen, the clinic physicians were free to leave, thereby incurring no wasted time. Perhaps the high rate of no-shows reflected patient awareness of these circumstances, but the habit presaged a problem if continued within the individualized appointment system of the Genesee Health Service.

Our observations showed that OPD clinics, particularly those that we have categorized as primary care, were used on a long-term, continuing basis. Of all visits, 72 percent were *revisits* by patients who had made at least one previous visit to the same clinic for treatment of the same general medical problem. Similarly, the visit disposition usually involved a follow-up appointment.

The data verified a great variation in physician staffing patterns among individual clinics, indicating not only differences in the qualifications of OPD physicians, but also the considerable complexities involved in managing the division as a single unit. Overall, 42 percent of the visits made during the two-week observation period were seen by attending physicians, 55 percent by house officers, and 2 percent by nurses only. For 1 percent of all visits no treatment was reported, because the person who made the visit voluntarily left without being seen by either a physician or a nurse.

The punctuality exhibited by physicians who served in the OPD during the study period left something to be desired. Approximately 30 percent of all OPD visits were made to clinic sessions that did not have a physician in attendance until at least fifteen minutes after the scheduled beginning of their session. Interestingly, house officers were no more punctual in their arrivals than were attending staff. Once the physician arrived, however, he was kept busy until the session was completed. Analysis indicated that a physician generally had at least one patient in an examination room during the entire clinic session.

The study verified that the periods patients spent waiting to be seen tended to be rather lengthy. The median waiting time for all clinic visits was forty-eight minutes, and approximately 20 percent of all visitors experienced waiting periods greater than ninety minutes. As would be expected, patient waiting times tended to increase when the clinic physician arrived late. We had assumed also that patients who themselves arrived late would have relatively short waiting times. This hypothesis was upheld; these patients neither had to wait for the physician to arrive, nor did they have to wait behind a long line of other patients.

Given the longer waiting times for early arrivers, we reasoned that return visitors would learn the "system" and react by arriving late. This hypothesis was not supported by the data. In fact, patients making return visits were significantly more likely to arrive on or before the appointed hour than were initial visitors. Three possible explanations are suggested:

1. Return visitors knew the hospital better and had less trouble finding the OPD area; or
2. Return visitors were more amenable and compliant; or
3. Return visitors did attempt to decrease their waiting time but, noting the first-come, first-served policy, mistakenly believed that coming early and getting in the front of the line would accomplish the goal.

Whatever their reason, for the most part, OPD patients were reasonably punctual. About 75 percent of all arrivals occurred within thirty minutes of the scheduled arrival times, and arrivals were as likely to be early as late.

The recorded lengths of time spent by patients in examination rooms (median: eighteen minutes), while only a rough approximation of time involved with providers, was an indication that patients were not unduly hurried through procedures and examinations. However, only in the maternity clinic did it appear that more time was taken with new patients than with return patients. In accord with our expectations, house staff generally spent a longer time with patients than did attending physicians, but our ability to control for "case mix" differences was quite limited.

Total waiting and examination time resulted in relatively lengthy visits to OPD. The median time between arrival and departure was sixty-eight minutes. The mean time of eighty-two minutes reflects the occurrence of some extremely long visits, which with the pattern of clinic scheduling created crowded conditions in the OPD area during peak periods in early morning and early afternoon. Yet the area was virtually empty at other times during the day.

The restricted scheduling of the various clinics obviously limited OPD's accessibility to patients. Most importantly, no procedure existed for responding to patient needs at night and on weekends, other than through the emergency room. Further, even during weekdays there appeared to be little opportunity for a patient to contact a physician by telephone, which for private patients is a customary means to acquire medical advice. Physicians remained in the OPD area only long enough to conduct their scheduled clinic sessions. The greatest part of their professional day was spent in private practice or in responsibilities elsewhere within the hospital.

Our interest in the accessibility of OPD services, and in the pattern of communications within the organization, led us to conduct a study of telephone utilization.[3] During a five-day period shortly after completion of the preceding collection of data, the nursing and clerical staffs were asked to categorize each incoming and outgoing telephone call, using a standardized format. A total of 737 calls, 472 incoming and 265 outgoing, were identified.

Results of the telphone study generally are not surprising. For example, calls to the hospital's medical records department were frequent. Further, a high volume of calls was recorded between OPD and the Genesee Health Service, which was assuming more and more of the patient load. Moreover, individual physicians were contacted frequently, reflecting the organizational effort required to operate a facility serviced by a large number of providers, none of whom is based there. Many of the outgoing calls were made simply to locate a particular doctor. Less expected was the finding that few calls were made between OPD and the Emergency Division. Thus, despite the overlap in the ED and OPD patient populations that we have documented, the data suggest little coordination of patient care.

Approximately one-third of all calls recorded during the study period were made by patients. Most of these concerned the scheduling of appointments. However, only ten appointment *cancellations* were recorded, which was a small portion of the total appointments not kept in any given week. Again we note the difficulties this pattern of patient behavior would create if manifested within an individualized appointment system. OPD staff apparently accepted this patient norm. We observed only one outgoing call to follow up a broken appointment.

Of major interest to us was the response to patients who called OPD seeking medical advice. Forty-nine requests for medical or drug-related information (as opposed to about 350 actual visits) were recorded during the week. Of this number, twenty-seven received some informational response, mostly from nurses, seven from physicians. The remainder were referred elsewhere or asked to schedule an appointment. Thus, the OPD structure appeared neither to encourage nor to provide adequate response to patient requests for such information.

The OPD staff were handicapped by obvious organizational barriers to communication. Yet, OPD functions were fulfilled, if not efficiently, at least with compassion, because of the small group of nurses, who provided ongoing coordinated care and advice to patients. While the physicians came and went, the nurses stayed. To a great extent, they countered the otherwise dispassionate character of the clinics. However, the basic problems of OPD did appear virtually insurmountable within the existing organizational structure. A new mode of care was required.

The Genesee Health Service

In contrast to the pervasive institutional setting that characterized the out-patient clinics, the Genesee Health Service was designed to create the intimacy and aesthetic appeal of a private group practice.[4] GHS patients use the same entrance and elevators as do the patients of other physicians in the building. The offices are decentralized into suites, each of which has its own waiting room and supporting staff. Administrative offices, a medical records area, a children's playroom, and a small laboratory are incorporated into the overall design, which won a local architectural award. The construction was funded in part by the OEO grant, in the amount of $250,000, and in part by the Hill-Burton program, in the amount of $100,000. In addition, OEO provided equipment funding of $84,000, and Genesee Hospital committed up to $100,000 for construction and equipment expenditures not covered by the grants.

GHS planners and the hospital board placed great emphasis on financial management.[5] Quite early in the transition period, a business manager was recruited and given charge of accounting and billing. Further, agreement was reached that relieved GHS of any fiscal responsibility for ancillary services rendered by other departments in the hospital. Also unlike OPD, fees competitive with private practitioners were charged, collection procedures followed, and discounts offered on an individual basis only to patients with demonstrated need. Expenses were watched closely, and allocations of indirect costs from the hospital were monitored to assure fairness and accuracy. Budgeting procedures, monthly income statements, and incentives for productivity also were instituted. All of these measures were implemented in accord with the conditions of the OEO grant, which also, in effect, guaranteed GHS reimbursement for any operating deficits incurred during the first several years of its existence. This contractual agreement was renewed on an annual basis from the Department of Health, Education, and Welfare, to which the grant was transferred when OEO was terminated.

It is GHS policy to accept a diversity of payment mechanisms, including fee-for-service, Medicare, and private insurance. A prepayment plan is offered through the Rochester Health Network (a corporate entity developed out of the Neighborhood Health Centers of Monroe County, Inc.),[6] and GHS physicians have participated in several foundation-type plans developed within the community. For Medicaid patients, GHS has replaced OPD as the hospital's outpatient facility. Accordingly, it receives a per-visit rate based on cost.

Arrangements for the provision of care generally are typical of any private group practice. Each patient is assigned a personal physician, and visits are made on an individualized appointment basis. Evening and Saturday office hours are available, and "on-call" coverage is provided at all other times.

GHS physicians are salaried employees of Genesee Hospital, although, as members of a distinct, organized medical group, they assume much of the responsibility for policy and operational decisions that affect their practice. Most of the members of the group are board-certified specialists in pediatrics or internal medicine, and they work full-time with GHS. Services in obstetrics/gynecology, the third major component, at first were provided through the hospital's existing residency program, to which later was added a full-time GHS specialist.[7]

The initial intent was to group GHS physicians into family-oriented teams. Each office suite was to be staffed by one or more teams each consisting of a pediatrician and an internist (and later an obstetrician), who would confer readily on problems relating to the family as a whole and thereby provide complete management of family care. This arrangement was tried, but it soon encountered difficulties. The need for joint consultations seldom arose. The provision of care in the new program was based on individual needs, and traditional family units were not as prevalent in the GHS patient population as had been anticipated. Moreover, elderly patients found the sometimes unrestrained presence of young children in the waiting room to be annoying. Most important were problems associated with the alternation of off-hour coverage among the specialists. After-hour patient needs often are preceived as urgent. The internists were uncomfortable in assuming responsibility for the treatment of children under these circumstances; similar discomfort attended the pediatricians when contacted by adult patients. Finally, the physicians identified strongly with their respective specialties and apparently preferred to align their patterns of communication accordingly. Consequently, the experiment with multispecialty suites lasted only three months, after which the suites were regrouped into separate specialties.

Although the model of a private group practice was emphasized in the development of the Genesee Health Service, several important differences should be mentioned. First, and most obvious, the medical group were committed to assume responsibility for care of the hospital's former outpatient population. Second, as part of the Department of Ambulatory Services, the group were particularly aware of the potential impact that they as primary-care physician might have in reducing "inappropriate" emergency-room use. Third, GHS affirmed a need for the creation of comprehensive services directed at the poor and, supported by the OEO grant, initiated a social services component to work closely with the medical group. Last, the staff endorsed the idea of community responsibility and supported the formation of an advisory board composed of provider, patient, and consumer representative.

Growth of the Program

We compiled and maintained a variety of statistics during the formative years of the Genesee Health Service.[8] We present some of these statistics here, in the belief that they provide a summary of program development and service utilization that will be useful to planners at other institutions. The period covered generally is the program's first 3½ years, updated by more recent information when available. The discussion relates only to services provided at the main center. Excluded are a satellite office that was opened in a suburban community and an off-site, established pediatric practice that affiliated briefly with GHS. These offices have influenced somewhat the overall development of the medical group, but they were not integral to the program or its basic objectives.

Physicians. The numbers of full-time-equivalent (FTE) physicians employed by the Genesee Health Service during the first 3½ years are shown in figure 4-1. At the end of this period, the great majority of physician services within pediatrics and medicine was being provided by practitioners employed in a full-time status, while the one full-time obstetrician/gynecologist represented approximately half of the resources available within that specialty. The medical group has continued to expand since these data were compiled. Recent (December 1979) data indicate the employment of 4.2 FTE pediatricians, 6.5 FTE internists and medical subspecialists, and 2.8 FTE ob/gyns.[9] In addition, GHS throughout the years has employed several nurse practitioners and physician assistants, who work under physician supervision but may have their own panels of patients and treat routine visits independently.

Visits. Figure 4-2 presents the monthly ambulatory visits made during the period of transition to GHS and, for comparison, to the OPD primary-care clinics. As shown, GHS utilization grew steadily. By the end of 3½ years, the new program was serving nearly five thousand visits a month. In fact, a slowing in the rate of growth at that time is attributable primarily to the physical limitations of the facility. Subsequently, additional office space was acquired on other floors of the professional building, and volume again increased. Table 4-1 presents the visit data in annual totals, including those of recent years.[10] Over eighty-four thousand visits now are being made to the Genesee Health Service each year.

Figure 4-3 portrays the ratio of monthly ambulatory visits per FTE physician, which can be viewed as a rough measure of productivity. For clarity, the full graph describes only the total practice, with the individual specialties represented at the far right by their respective ratios at the end of the study period. The overall trend is rather erratic but generally upward, as would be expected. The relatively high productivity in pediatrics is consis-

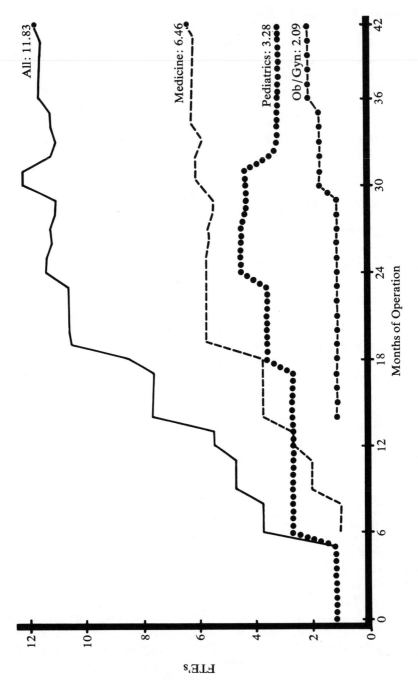

Figure 4-1. Full-Time-Equivalent Physicians

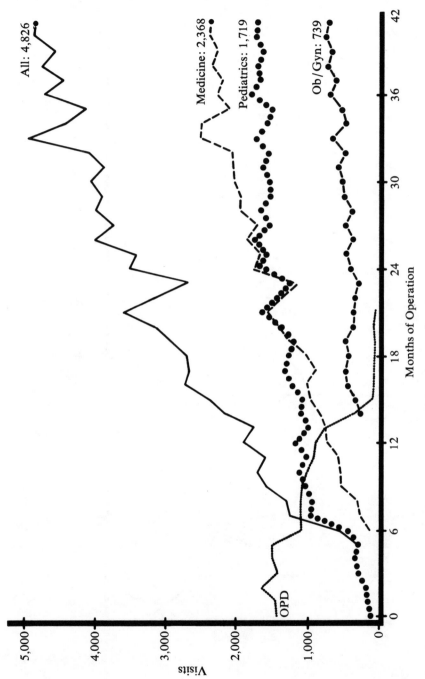

Figure 4-2. Monthly Visits

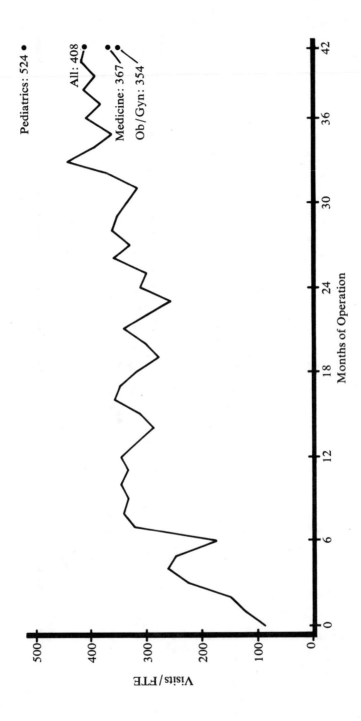

Figure 4-3. Physician Productivity

Table 4-1
GHS Ambulatory Visits, 1972–1979

Year	Pediatrics	Medicine	Ob/Gyn	Total
1972	6,902	2,387	–	9,289
1973	15,081	12,960	3,754	31,795
1974	19,048	23,329	5,506	47,883
1975	20,535	31,426	9,004	60,965
1976	22,942	33,354	6,316	62,612
1977	26,424	38,521	12,048	76,993
1978	27,265	39,339	12,098	78,702
1979	31,810	40,320	12,005	84,135

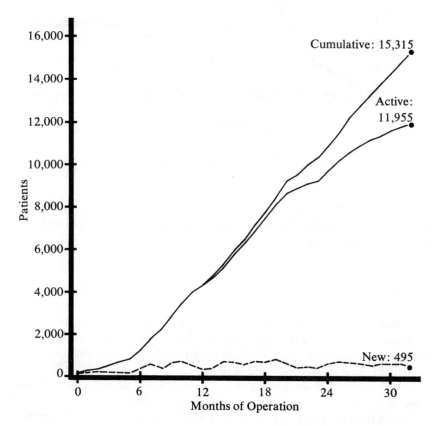

Figure 4-4. Patient Population

tent with figures 4–1 and 4–2, which show that the practice had stabilized somewhat by that point. Further, pediatric visits generally require less physician time than visits made to internal medicine, thereby enabling each practitioner to see a greater number. Ob/gyn visits generally are also less

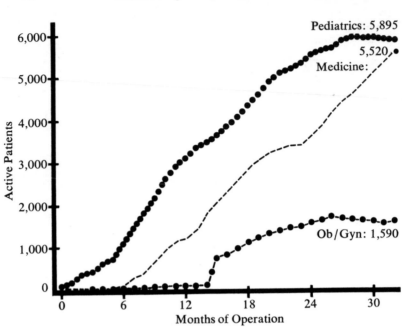

Figure 4-5. Active Patient Population

time-consuming, but, because the obstetricians spend greater portions of their workday on deliveries and inpatient work, they are less available for office visits and therefore show relatively low productivity in ambulatory care.

Patients. While counts of visits are useful and a readily available measure of services rendered by GHS, we state earlier our belief that the number of individual patients seen is the more important indicator of impact on the community. To obtain this information, during the thirty-third month of GHS operation, we selected a systematic (one out of every fifteen) sample of patient medical records and abstracted their patterns of utilization. Unlike the OPD-ED samples of visits, the GHS sample of records yielded without further adjustment a representative group of patients.

With the use of three trend lines, figure 4-4 shows the estimated growth of the GHS patient population. Judging from the bottom line on the graph, new patients were introduced to GHS at a relatively constant rate of about five hundred per month. The upper line of *cumulative patients* shows the number of new patients seen cumulatively up to and including each month. Thus, through the thirty-third month of its existence, approximately fifteen thousand patients had been treated at GHS.

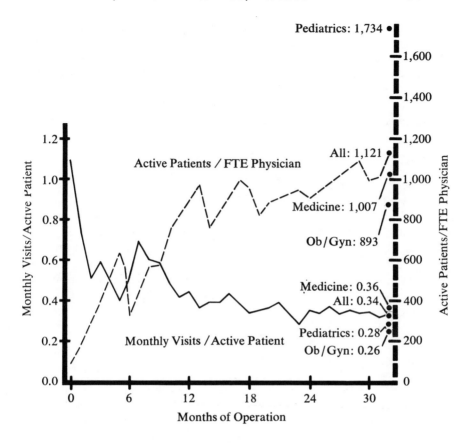

Figure 4-6. Patient Load and Visit Frequency

The number of cumulative patients is not adjusted for transient use and other departures from the practice and therefore is deceiving in terms of patient load. Accordingly, we defined an *active patient* for any given month as a patient who either (1) had made at least one GHS visit during the previous twelve months, or (2) had made a visit only prior to the most recent twelve-month period but made a later visit between the month of interest and the date of the sample selection. The middle line of figure 4-4 shows the growth of the active patient population. Figure 4-5 provides active patient trends for each of the three specialities. While the pediatric and ob/gyn practices appear to have leveled off by the thirty-third month, the internal medicine practice shows continued growth.

Ratios of active patients per FTE physician were computed as a second indicator of productivity. Figure 4-6 shows that this trend was generally upward. The three specialties exhibit differences similiar to those observed for "visits per FTE." Figure 4-6 also shows the trend in monthly visits per active patient. The flattening of this line suggests the validity of our definition of an active patient. Further, the last month's overall average of 4.1 visits per patient per year (obtained by multiplying the calculated monthly ratio of .34 by 12) compares reasonably with national data. Observe also that the two ratios of figure 4-6 relate closely to figure 4-3. Formally, monthly visits per FTE physician equal active patients per FTE physician multiplied by monthly visits per active patient. Thus, if physician productivity is at issue, the use of patient statistics may provide helpful clarification.

With the large increases in GHS physician manpower and visit volume that have taken place in the years since our study, it is certain that the GHS patient population also has increased greatly. We assume that our last calculated ratio of .34 monthly visits per active patient is reasonably stable and divide it into 7,011 — the average number of monthly visits made to GHS during the 1979 — to derive a population of 20,620 active patients projected to 1979. Although this projection is only a rough approximation, it illustrates the remarkable growth that has been experienced by GHS during its first seven years.

Notes

1. Two useful summaries of the literature on hospital outpatient clinics are Michael M. Stewart and Charles H. Goodrich, "Special Problems of Primary Care in Large Urban Hospitals," in *Community Hospitals and the Challenge of Primary Care*, edited by John H. Bryant et al. (New York: Center for Community Health Systems, Columbia University, 1975), pp. 105-122; and Steven Jonas and Barbara Rimer, "Ambulatory Care," in *Health Care Delivery in the United States*, ed. by Steven Jonas (New York: Springer Publishing Company, 1977), pp. 120-163.

2. Detailed procedures, data, and analysis are available from the authors in Ralph Ullman, "Genesee Outpatient Division Study I: Patient Flow," mimeographed (Rochester, N.Y.: Health Services Research Center, The Genesee Hospital, 1973).

3. Ralph Ullman, "Genesee Outpatient Division Study II: Telephone Communications," mimeographed (Rochester, N.Y.: Health Services Research Center, The Genesee Hospital, 1973).

4. For other descriptions of the Genesee Health Service, see James A. Block, "Hospital Innovations in the Community: Ambulatory Care," *Bulletin of the New York Academy of Medicine* 55(1979):104; Seth B. Goldsmith, "Organizing for Primary Care in Community Hospitals: Five Examples," in *Community Hospitals and the Challenge of Primary Care*,

Bryant et al., pp. 81–103; and Chris Bale, "Can Physicians' Groups Carry the Outpatient Load for Hospitals?" *Group Practice* vol. 26, no. 2 (March-April 1977):8. For a comprehensive review of the literature and issues related to this form of organization, see Stephen J. Williams et al., "Hospital-Sponsored Primary Care Group Practices: A Developing Modality of Care," *Health and Medical Care Services Review* vol. 1, no. 516 (September-December 1978):1.

5. For details on the procedures of financial management instituted within the Genesee Health Service, see Marshall V. Rozzi, "Fiscal Planning of Changes in Ambulatory Care," in *Community Hospitals*, Bryant, pp. 143–162.

6. Donna Regenstreif et al., "Prepayment and the Genesee Health Service," *Medical Group Management* vol. 26, no. 6 (November-December 1979):38.

7. Robert C. Tatelbaum and Donna I. Regenstreif, "An Ambulatory Model for an Obstetrics and Gynecology Residency Program," *Journal of Medical Education* 53 (1978):344.

8. Ralph Ullman, "Utilization and Growth of the Genesee Health Service, 1972–1975," mimeographed (Rochester, N.Y.: Health Services Research Center, The Genesee Hospital, 1975).

9. Glenn Gravino, Genesee Health Service, personal communication.

10. Ibid.

5 Impact of the Genesee Health Service

The planners of the Genesee Health Service believed that the deficiencies generally associated with hospital outpatient settings owed fundamentally to the absence of any single physician from a position to assume the responsibility for the ongoing management of patient care. Clearly, continuity of care in any primary-care facility is enhanced greatly by a full-time staff of highly motivated physicians, and the recruitment of such staff was a major administrative objective. While there was good reason to believe that organizational attributes of the program, such as the close hospital affiliation and the group-practice atmosphere, would favorably influence prospective candidates,[1] these factors in themselves were not considered sufficient to assure acquisition of the desired personnel.

Observers of the frustrations experienced by physicians involved in a comprehensive-care program directed at low-income patients have concluded that "no mortal physician can be asked to care for low-income groups exclusively for an indefinite time.[2] A good part of the satisfaction that physicians derive from their work comes from seeing their patients benefit from their ministrations. Yet, prognoses for inner-city patients generally are poor. Patient problems often are compounded by social circumstances, over which neither they nor their physicians have any control. Consequently, GHS planners perceived that the recruitment and retention of a team of highly motivated physicians would require a much broader-based patient population than was characteristic of the hospital's outpatient clinics. Relaxation of OEO's customary requirements for the proportion of non-poor that could be served by a funded network was an important concession that allowed GHS planners to pursue this objective.

To Genesee planners, the ultimate acquisition of a broad socioeconomic mix of patients was seen as the most important prerequisite to the creation of a viable, satisfying "one-class" system of care, which, in turn, was viewed as the best way to improve the care rendered to the low-income, clinic patients whose circumstances were of primary concern. The technical quality of care per se was not a specific focus of the program, nor was there any expectation that the Genesee Health Service would create a measurable change in the health status of its patient population, at least during the short duration of the research project. More central to the goals of program developers were acquisition and retention of the desired patient population, improvements in the accessibility and continuity of care, creation of attitudinal changes consonant with the norms of the practice, and the financial viability of the overall endeavor. To these issues we now focus our attention.

The Patient Population

Table 5-1 shows the estimated numbers of individual patients served by GHS during the twelve-month period prior to the date of selection of the patient sample, which we describe in chapter 4. Defined thus, the GHS patient population can be compared directly to the primary-care population of OPD, which we present earlier (see table 3–10). We observe that, although only thirty-three months old, the GHS specialities of pediatrics and medicine already were serving a patient population over twice as large as OPD had served. At the time, the ob/gyn population had not increased, but an interesting difference is apparent. Patients in the GHS ob/gyn practice were much more likely also to have made a *medical* visit during the same year, which suggests the effect of an emphasis on comprehensive care and better coordination among the GHS specialties.

GHS Utilization

Table 5–2 provides an estimated breakdown by visit frequency of the defined GHS patient population. The resulting pattern of utilization indicates that the bulk of services were rendered to patients who received continuing care at the facility. Only 10 percent of the total visits in the designated twelve-month period were made by individuals who made but one visit.

Table 5-1
Estimated GHS Patient Population, 10/6/73-10/6/74

Specialty		Estimated Patients
Pediatrics		5,745
Internal Medicine		5,490
Ob/Gyn		1,440
Obstetrics	420	
Gynecology	1,200	
(Less: both)	(180)	
(Less: pediatrics and ob/gyn)		(45)
(Less: medicine and ob/gyn)		(630)
Total		12,000

Other Genesee Utilization

The estimated utilization of all Genesee Hospital services by the GHS patient population is shown in table 5-3. Compared with the OPD population these data show slightly lower rates of inpatient utilization. The moderately higher total number of admissions and inpatient-days is attributed to the much larger population size. Emergency-room utilization was much lower among GHS patients, a subject to which we devote attention later in this chapter.

Patient Characteristics

Table 5-4 presents a comparison of the GHS and OPD populations using the limited sociodemographic information available in patient charts. Judging from the source of payment, GHS did attract a different patient population. Clinic patients predominantly were eligible for Medicaid, GHS patients predominantly were not. This change, however, was not the consequence of a loss of Medicaid patients. On the contrary, we estimate that over nine hundred more Medicaid patients were seen in GHS than in the primary care clinics, during the years compared.

A comparison on the basis of geographic area of residence (table 5-5) shows that, with one exception, GHS substantially increased the numbers of

Table 5-2
Estimated GHS Utilization by Specialty, 10/6/73-10/6/74

Year's Visits Within Specialty	Pediatrics		Medicine		Ob/Gyn		All Specialties[a]	
	Patients	Visits	Patients	Visits	Patients	Visits	Patients	Visits
1	1,950 (34%)	1,950 (11%)	1,935 (35%)	1,935 (10%)	615 (43%)	615 (13%)	4,080 (34%)	4,080 (10%)
2	1,260 (22%)	2,520 (14%)	945 (17%)	1,890 (10%)	240 (17%)	480 (10%)	2,190 (18%)	4,380 (10%)
3	870 (15%)	2,610 (15%)	660 (12%)	1,980 (10%)	195 (14%)	585 (13%)	1,605 (13%)	4,815 (12%)
4-6	1,080 (19%)	5,055 (29%)	1,155 (21%)	5,580 (29%)	225 (16%)	1,125 (24%)	2,475 (21%)	11,910 (29%)
7+	585 (10%)	5,520 (31%)	795 (14%)	8,070 (41%)	165 (11%)	1,815 (39%)	1,650 (14%)	16,545 (40%)
Totals	5,745 (100%)	17,655 (100%)	5,490 (100%)	19,455 (100%)	1,440 (100%)	4,620 (100%)	12,000 (100%)	41,730 (100%)

[a]In this and subsequent tables, the data presented for all specialties are not the sums of the data related to the individual specialties, because some patients made visits to more than one specialty (see table 5-1).

Table 5-3
Estimated Utilization of Hospital Services by GHS
Patients, 10/6/74-10/6/75

	Pediatrics	*Medicine*	*Ob/Gyn*	*All*
Patients	5,745	5,490	1,440	12,000
GHS visits within specialty	17,655	19,455	4,620	41,730
Per patient	3.1	3.5	3.2	3.5
Other GHS visits	135	2,040	2,475	—
Per patient	0.0	0.4	1.7	—
Percentage of patients with at least one visit	1%	11%	47%	—
Dental, eye, and surgical clinic visits	735	1,530	180	2,325
Per patient	0.1	0.3	0.1	0.2
Percentage of patients with at least one visit	4%	8%	4%	6%
Emergency division visits	1,935	3,750	1,635	6,285
Per patient	0.3	0.7	1.1	0.5
Percentage of patients with at least one visit	25%	36%	49%	31%
Inpatient admissions	255	1,020	480[a]	1,485
Per patient	0.0	0.2	0.3	0.1
Percentage of patients with at least one admission	4%	14%	31%	10%
Average stay (days) per admission	7.0	8.8	5.8	7.6
Total inpatient-days	1,785	8,955	2,760	11,280

[a]Includes 300 obstetric admissions.

residents in each geographic area who looked to the hospital for their primary care. The exception is the area of center A, a neighborhood health center that had been established well before GHS. The extensive area served by GHS clearly does not fit the model of a geographically focused program. While the capture rate of patients was highest in the area immediately surrounding the hospital, it was only moderately higher than rates found in other areas.

Sources of Patients

Previous Genesee Utilization

The extent to which all GHS patients (not just the defined twelve-months' population) had utilized other Genesee Hospital services prior to their first GHS visit is presented in table 5-6. We estimate that 22 percent of all GHS patients had made a recent primary-care clinic visit, 33 percent a prior OPD

Table 5-4
OPD-GHS Patient Sociodemographic Comparisons
(percent)

	Pediatrics		Medicine		Ob/Gyn		All	
	OPD	GHS	OPD	GHS	OPD	GHS	OPD	GHS
Sex								
Male	58	52	40	38	—	—	39	42
Female	42	48	60	62	100	100	61	58
Age								
0-9	89	81	3	0	0	0	39	39
10-19	11	19	13	12	26	20	16	16
20-29	0	0	20	32	52	54	9	19
30-39	0	0	15	16	13	17	8	8
40-49	0	0	15	13	4	6	6	7
50-59	0	0	17	12	3	1	7	6
60-69	0	0	9	7	1	0	3	3
70-79	0	0	5	4	1	1	2	2
80+	0	0	3	3	0	1	1	1
Race/ethnicity								
White	58	59	60	64	50	59	57	61
Black	42	37	40	32	50	37	43	35
Spanish-speaking[a]	—	4	—	4	—	4	—	4
Source of payment								
Medicaid	66	46	63	32	72	51	65	39
Other third party[b]	25	47	26	55	15	34	24	50
No third party	10	7	11	13	13	15	12	11

Note: Columns may not sum to 100 percent because of rounding.

[a]Not categorized for the OPD sample.

[b]Includes any medical coverage, not necessarily ambulatory only.

Table 5-5
OPD-GHS Patient Residence Comparison

Area	Population (1970)	Estimated Patients OPD			GHS		(%) (Patients/1000)
Rochester health network							
Genesee Health Service	44,980	1,232	(21%)	(27)	2,370	(20%)	(53)
Center A	22,218	821	(14%)	(37)	780	(7%)	(35)
Center B	61,252	1,793	(30%)	(29)	2,445	(20%)	(40)
Center C	81,007	1,242	(21%)	(15)	2,550	(21%)	(31)
Other Rochester	86,776	411	(7%)	(5)	1,170	(10%)	(13)
Southeast suburbs	132,536	170	(3%)	(1)	1,110	(9%)	(8)
Other	—	220	(4%)	—	1,575	(13%)	—

visit of any type, 54 percent a prior ambulatory visit, either OPD or ED, and 64 percent some previous encounter, either ambulatory or inpatient.

Two problems obtain with respect to a comparison of GHS patients who had made a recent primary-care clinic visit with the OPD primary-care population. First, the time periods are not strictly comparable. The OPD estimates are based on utilization within a predetermined year, while the GHS figures are partly open-ended, depending on the date of each patient's first GHS visit. Second, an evaluative judgment about the successful retention of the primary-care clinic population is not possible without more information about mobility, maturation, health changes, and other factors that influence the likelihood of a person's continued use of a health-care facility over a long period of time.

Former Private Practices

Two of the first full-time GHS physicians, an internist and a pediatrician, had private practices in Rochester before joining the program. Based on a separate review of medical records, we estimate that about seven hundred

Table 5-6
GHS Patients' Previous Genesee Hospital Utilization

	Estimated Patients (%)			
	Pediatrics	Medicine	Ob/Gyn	All
Cumulative Patients to 10/6/74	7,740 (100%)	6,735 (100%)	2,010 (100%)	15,345 (100%)
Primary-Care Clinic visit since 1/1/71	1,440 (19%)	1,530 (23%)	915 (46%)	3,330 (22%)
Other previous OPD visit	1,440 (19%)	2,100 (31%)	810 (40%)	3,810 (25%)
Any OPD visit	2,190 (20%)	2,520 (37%)	1,110 (55%)	5,100 (33%)
ED visit	3,210 (41%)	4,035 (60%)	1,440 (72%)	7,830 (51%)
Any ambulatory visit	3,375 (44%)	4,275 (63%)	1,590 (79%)	8,355 (54%)
Born at Genesee	2,490 (32%)	210 (3%)	105 (5%)	2,715 (18%)
Inpatient admission	780 (10%)	2,445 (36%)	1,005 (50%)	3,555 (23%)
Inpatient, including newborn	2,970 (38%)	2,535 (38%)	1,005 (50%)	5,835 (38%)
Any inpatient or ambulatory encounter	4,575 (59%)	4,485 (67%)	1,620 (81%)	9,780 (64%)

GHS patients were transfers from these two practices. It is likely that word-of-mouth referrals from this core group of nonclinic patients had an influence on the growth of the program.

Patient Behavior

It is evident that during the period of our research the Genesee Health Service experienced substantial growth. For one reason or another, most of these patients were familiar with Genesee as a source of care. Many came from what we have defined as the hospital's outpatient primary-care population. But it is clear also that the basic constituency had broadened, and that the health-service population had become more representative of the community as a whole.

The goal of creating a one-class system of care was motivated partly by normative values of social justice, and partly because of the belief that only in such a practice setting would efforts to improve the well-being of low-income patients have much chance of success. Planners at Genesee hoped that clinic patients, once introduced to the administrative and clinical norms of the primary-care group practice, would begin to acquire different values about health care. It was reasoned that, in time, these patients would develop confidence in their doctors and become comfortable in the new practice setting. Planners believed that these predicted changes in attitude would have a favorable impact on patient behavior. They hypothesized such effects as improved compliance, more frequent use of the telephone to obtain medical advice, and reduced use of the emergency room. In short, they believed that patients would become more disciplined and efficient in the use of health-care resources. In this section, we report the results of several studies that were designed to test these hypotheses.

Telephone Utilization

Data for a study of telephone communication in the Genesee Health Service were collected during a seven-day period in March 1974.[3] Additional information was obtained from the medical group's answering service, which referred off-hour calls to the physicians responsible for coverage. A total of approximately two thousand incoming calls were received during the study period.

The major reasons for the conduct of the study were to document the services provided to patients over the telephone by the GHS medical staff and to investigate the utilization of these services by the patient population. For the week studied, 456 telephone "encounters" were recorded, most with a physician, some with a pediatric nurse practitioner, or a physician's associate in internal medicine. The number of telephone encounters was approximately half the number of visits made to the facility during the week. Thus, telephone accessibility does appear to be an important aspect of GHS service. And, clearly, this opportunity for patient-provider communication was a great improvement over that observed in OPD and reported in the previous chapter.

Telephone encounters between providers and the parents of pediatric patients were more numerous than those recorded with adult patients. Whether this was the consequence of the relative maturity of the pediatric practice, or a greater emphasis placed by the pediatrician on this form of utilization, or simply an increased likelihood of parents to phone because of greater concern and uncertainty about their children's ailments, could not be ascertained from this study. The findings, however, do correspond closely to the reported views of patients, which we discuss in chapter 6.

Emergency-Room Utilization

It was hoped that by providing continuity of care and by making physicians more accessible through telephone communication, patients would become less dependent on the emergency room, and that such utilization would be reduced. The anticipated reduction was to be effected primarily through the transfer to GHS of the former clinic patients, whose frequent use of the emergency room we have documented. It was expected also that overall emergency-room use over time would be reduced by follow-up referrals to GHS of emergency-room patients who reported no source of primary care, and by direct triage to GHS of these patients when their visits to the emergency room were for nonurgent problems. However, as the program developed, the last approach was employed only infrequently, because of the difficulties encountered in fitting walk-in visits into the appointment schedules of GHS physicians.

In assessing the impact of GHS on emergency-room use at Genesee, we were faced with several methodological problems. First, and most important, we did not have a controlled setting. A change in the population base or the creation of other local new ambulatory facilities also might have affected utilization of Genesee's Emergency Division. Further, the relevant population base itself was undefined. As we show earlier, patients came to GHS and to ED from a diversity of geographic areas. Thus the technique of ascertaining change in the volume of emergency-room visits originating from a particular area, which had been employed in several studies of the effects of neighborhood health centers,[4] was not appropriate to our situation. Because of these structural problems, we decided that no single analytic design would yield definite conclusions. Instead, we looked for consistent trends resulting from three separate analyses. First, we compared the volume of ED visits made in 1971 (prior to development of GHS) with the volume made in 1974 (after GHS development). Second, we compared the estimated ED utilization of the OPD primary-care population with that of the comparable twelve-months' sample of GHS patients. Third, for the full GHS sample, we compared the frequency of ED utilization by patients before their first GHS visits with that by the same patients after their first GHS visits.[5]

1971 versus 1974. Table 5-7 presents the numbers of visits made to the Genesee Emergency Division in the years between 1971 and 1974, to those specialties the utilization of which the Genesee Health Service might be expected to affect. We observe that these specialties accounted for less than half of the ED's total utilization, even in 1971. Nevertheless, the nearly 50-percent reduction of pediatric visits between 1971 and 1974 is striking. The question is: how much of the reduction can be attributed to the use of alternative facilities? During this period, the number of births in the Rochester area decreased by 19 percent, a factor that in itself should have reduced substantially the demand for emergency-room services by young children.

We made two estimates of the independent effect of the lowered birth rate on pediatric ED utilization. First, we took a visits-by-age distribution, which had been estimated in the base-line utilization study, adjusted it for cohorts of area births in subsequent years, and derived an expected reduction in pediatric ED visits of 18 percent. Alternatively, we examined children's use of ED surgical services, which had been listed separately at Genesee. Assuming that the observed reduction of 13 percent between 1971 and 1974 reflected primarily the impact of the changed population base, we anticipated the same 13 percent reduction in pediatric visits. Employing these estimates as upper and lower bounds of the birth rate's effect leaves a

Table 5-7
Emergency-Room Visits, 1971-1974

	1971	1972	1973	1974	Change 1971-1974 Visits (%)
Pediatrics	6,604	5,804	4,077	3,372	− 3,232 (− 49%)
Medicine	11,509	11,495	11,736	12,198	+ 689 (+ 6%)
Ob/Gyn	2,314	2,366	2,146	1,959	− 355 (− 15%)
Other[a]	23,368	23,623	23,971	23,024	− 344 (− 1%)
Total	43,795	43,288	41,930	40,553	− 3,242 (− 7%)

Note: Excluded are employee visits, scheduled visits, and arrivals for which no services were provided.
[a]Dental, eye, ENT, genito-urinary, orthopedic, and surgical.

31–35 percent reduction to be accounted for by other factors, of which GHS was likely to be the major influence.

Table 5-7 shows no substantial change in adult use of the emergency room. The volume of medical visits remained essentially constant, the slight increase being the result of additional psychiatric visits attracted by the hospital's new community mental-health center. The moderate percentage decrease in ob/gyn visits was of little importance, because of the small volume generated in that specialty. But the decrease cannot be attributed to the lowered birth rate, since few of these visits were related to pregnancies.

OPD versus GHS. Comparisons of emergency-room utilization between the OPD primary-care population and the GHS patients are made in table 5–8. Because the two populations are quite different in composition, we examine only differences in utilization among Medicaid patients. The greatest difference is apparent in pediatrics. GHS pediatric patients made substant-

Table 5-8
Emergency-Room Utilization by OPD and GHS Patients

Utilization	Pediatrics		Medicine		Ob/Gyn		All	
	OPD	GHS	OPD	GHS	OPD	GHS	OPD	GHS
All Patients								
$(n)^a$	(127)	(383)	(106)	(366)	(79)	(96)	(295)	(800)
Estimated patients	2,563	5,745	2,128	5,490	1,538	1,440	5,890	12,000
Estimated ED users	1,468	1,425	1,380	1,995	849	705	3,447	3,735
Estimated ED visits	2,997	1,935	3,456	3,750	2,420	1,635	7,857	6,285
Percent ED users	57%	25%^{b}	65%	36%^{b}	55%	49%	59%	31%^{b}
ED visits/ED user	2.0	1.4^c	2.5	1.9^c	2.9	2.3	2.3	1.7^c
ED visits/patient	1.2	0.3^c	1.6	0.7^c	1.6	1.1	1.3	0.5^c
Medicaid Only								
$(n)^a$	(77)	(177)	(62)	(117)	(54)	(49)	(178)	(315)
Estimated patients	1,679	2,655	1,333	1,755	1,104	735	3,813	4,725
Estimated ED users	1,186	825	943	975	685	420	2,582	1,935
Estimated ED visits	2,614	1,110	2,505	2,295	2,065	1,155	6,339	3,660
Percent ED users	71%	31%^{b}	71%	56%^{b}	62%	57%	68%	41%^{b}
ED visits/ED user	2.2	1.3^c	2.7	2.4	3.0	2.8	2.5	1.9^c
ED visits/patient	1.6	0.4^c	1.9	1.3^c	1.9	1.6	1.7	0.8^c

[a]The OPD *n*'s are adjusted so as to correct for the different probabilities of sampling patients from a visit universe. The process yields a total of "cases" much less than the number of visits actually sampled, hence the results reported for the significance tests are conservative.

[b]$p \le$, 05, chi-square for difference in proportions, one-tailed.

[c]$p \le$, 05, Student's *t* for difference in means, one-tailed.

ially less use of the emergency room, based on all three measures employed in the analysis. In medicine, the differences are not as great, although statistically significant in two of the three measures. Little difference is apparent among ob/gyn Medicaid patients.

The OPD-GHS comparisons are deficient in two respects. First, by restricting the samples to Medicaid patients we are not likely to create perfectly comparable populations. Numerous distinctions still may differentiate the two groups and be at least partially responsible for the observed difference in utilization, although further controls using other sociodemographic variables yielded no results that conflict with those presented. Second, the data are only visit totals, which do not reflect the timing of the visits within the defined periods and therefore may be misleading. Thus, if a facility provided a relatively greater volume of follow-up care for emergency-room visits, the utilization statistics of its patients would be inflated. The third analysis, which compares the utilization patterns of the same individuals in two different time periods, avoids both of these problems, although the possibility of multiple causation remains.

GHS Patients: Before versus After. Annualized rates of ED utilization by GHS patients before and after their first GHS encounters are presented in table 5-9. In addition to the breakdown by specialty, we make two further separations of the data. First, the ED visits are divided into those resulting from an accidental injury (over which GHS would be expected to have relatively less effect), and those not related to accidents. Second, patients are categorized according to whether or not they had made a recent visit to the primary-care clinics, before their first use of GHS. The data show the importance of these distinctions. While the composite mean rate of ED utilization by GHS patients decreased significantly after their first encounters with the new program, major differences by specialty are apparent once again. Further, the overall reduction is attributable primarily to a large decrease in utilization by former clinic patients. As expected, ED visits related to accidental injury were not lessened.

The data on pediatrics reinforces the earlier findings about the effectiveness of this specialty in reducing emergency-room utilization. The estimated difference in annualized rates among former clinic users represents a reduction of 63 percent, almost one visit per year. Even among children new to the hospital's outpatient facilities, a statistically significant reduction in nonaccident visits is observed. Recognizing that these results could be a function of the maturation of the pediatric population during the period studied, we examined utilization rates for children of different ages, but we found no consistent relationship. We conclude that maturation was at most a minor factor compared to use of GHS.

Results regarding adult utilization are mixed. For former clinic patients

Table 5-9
GHS Patients' Emergency-Room Utilization

Utilization	Pediatrics			Medicine			Ob/Gyn			All		
	Former OPD (n = 96)	Others (420)	All (516)	Former OPD (102)	Others (347)	All (449)	Former OPD (61)	Others (73)	All (134)	Former OPD (222)	Others (801)	All (1023)
Accidents												
Mean post-GHS ED visits/year	.16	.09	.10	.17	.13	.14	.15	.22	.19	.17	.11	.12
Mean pre-GHS ED visits/year	.18	.08	.10	.29	.11	.15	.16	.09	.12	.21	.09	.12
Difference[a]	(.02)	.00	(.00)	(.12)[c]	.03	(.01)	(.00)	.14	.07	(.05)	.02	.01
Estimated yearly visits[a,b] increase (decrease)	(31)	24	(6)	(182)	134	(48)	(4)	150	146	(155)	274	118
Nonaccidents												
Mean post-GHS ED visits/year	.35	.18	.22	.76	.31	.41	.89	.71	.79	.58	.25	.32
Mean pre-GHS ED visits/year	1.21	.32	.49	1.06	.27	.45	.88	.27	.55	1.09	.30	.47
Difference[a]	(.86)[c]	(.14)[c]	(.27)[c]	(.30)[c]	.04	(.04)	.01	.44	.24	(.50)[c]	(.05)	(.15)[c]
Estimated yearly visits[a,b] increase (decrease)	(1233)	(878)	(2111)	(459)	193	(267)	12	478	490	(1678)	(631)	(2308)
All Visits												
Mean post-GHS ED visits/year	.51	.27	.31	.93	.44	.55	1.05	.93	.99	.75	.36	.45
Mean pre-GHS ED visits/year	1.39	.40	.59	1.35	.38	.60	1.04	.36	.67	1.30	.39	.59
Difference[a]	(.88)[c]	(.14)	(.27)[c]	(.42)[c]	.06	(.05)	.01	.57	.32	(.55)[c]	(.03)	(.14)[c]
Estimated yearly visits[a,b] increase (decrease)	(1263)	(854)	(2117)	(642)	327	(315)	8	628	636	(1834)	(357)	(2190)

Note: Portions of this table were presented in Ralph Ullman et. al., "Impact of a Primary Care Group Practice on Emergency Room Utilization at a Community Hospital," *Medical Care* 16 (1978): 723.

[a]Computed prior to rounding of visits/year rates.

[b]"Difference" $\times n \times 15$ (where 15 is the inverse of the sampling ratio).

[c] ... ted t test for difference in means, one-tailed.

in the GHS medical specialty, a statistically significant reduction in ED utilization is noted, but a slight per capita increase among the larger number of patients not seen previously in OPD substantially limited the overall impact of this specialty. Among ob/gyn patients, GHS apparently did not change emergency-room use in the desired direction. ED utilization by former clinic patients remained essentially the same; by other ob/gyn patients, utilization actually increased. We conclude that the modest decrease in total yearly ob/gyn ED visits indicated in table 5-7 is attributable most likely to factors other than the Genesee Health Service.

Because of the growth of GHS during the period studied, the increases (decreases) in yearly visits estimated in table 5-9 cannot be considered precise estimates of the impact of the new program during a particular year. These figures, however, are useful in illustrating the relative extent to which each specialty and patient group contributed to an overall effect. Viewed in this manner, the total net saving of 2,190 ED visits is attributable, almost entirely, to the GHS pediatric practice.

Summary and Discussion. A reasonably clear pattern emerges from the three analyses. The Genesee Health Service appears to have had a substantial effect on parents' use of the Genesee emergency room for their children. We estimate conservatively a reduction of two thousand annual visits, or approximately 30 percent of the former pediatric ED volume. GHS also appears to have been successful in reducing emergency-room utilization among those adults who characteristically depended on hospital ambulatory services. The overall impact on adult utilization of the Emergency Division seems negligible, however, because of higher rates of use among new patients attracted to the hospital. The GHS ob/gyn practice probably had little or no favorable impact, which we attribute to the relative similarity between its organization and the former OPD structure during the period of study. Unfortunately we could not evaluate the effect of the subsequent full-time GHS affiliation by a board-certified obstetrician/gynecologist.

The apparent effect of the GHS pediatric group is impressive and most encouraging. From these findings, as well as those reported by a neighborhood health center in Rochester,[6] we conclude that new primary-care services can provide acceptable alternatives to pediatric emergency-room use and that, in one urban area at least, this has been accomplished successfully. Also encouraging are the utilization patterns of the former OPD users, adults as well as children, which provide evidence that the provision of a personalized source of primary care can influence patients to modify their behavior.

Within the longitudinal analysis of ED utilization by GHS patients, *increased* rates are found among adults not seen previously in OPD. This result reminds us that our data come only from one hospital, and it does not imply necessarily an increase in *total* emergency-room use by these patients. The GHS population may have included some individuals who previously had used other emergency rooms in the area but by then considered Genesee to be their source of all ambulatory care, "emergency" or otherwise. While the increased use of ED that would result from this effect appears to have been dominated by countervailing forces in pediatrics, this was not so apparently among adult patients. Thus, we speculate that a hospital-based program that attracts new ambulatory patients may expand overall use of the hospital's facilities to the point where its own emergency room realizes little net reduction in utilization, even if community-wide use has lessened.

We stress earlier the importance of the initial pattern of ambulatory utilization at Genesee. Our studies indicate that ED was used as a "family doctor" by only a small proportion of its patients. Further, the primary-care population served in the outpatient clinics was not a large one. Thus, opportunity for the new primary-care group practice to create a major change in overall emergency-room utilization patterns appears quite limited. Even the estimated reduction of two thousand pediatric ED visits—when viewed as about six fewer visits per day—is not large enough to effect any major change in staffing patterns.

Partly because of our findings, Genesee administrators became convinced that the new group practice would not evolve into a panacea for the overburdened emergency room. Consequently, a restructuring was conducted within the Emergency Division itself. Two separate areas were created: one for truly emergent cases and one for less urgent visits. Using a triage approach,[7] ED arrivals now are directed toward that area in which care can be rendered with the more appropriate degree of privacy, medical expertise, and support facilities. With the Genesee Health Service continuing as an integral unit of the Department of Ambulatory Services, the hospital now provides a set of facilities that appear to meet differentially the range of demands expressed by the Rochester community.

Preventive Care in Pediatrics

The provision of comprehensive health services to the children of indigent families in Rochester was an important objective of the Genesee Health Service. Inner-city health care for the poor is hampered by a complex set of social, economic, and geographical barriers. Whether these families would utilize the services of personal physicians in the same way as do families more accustomed to such arrangements was uncertain. To study this question, we directed our attention to infants delivered by staff obstetricians at Genesee.[8] These children appeared particularly at risk of not receiving essential immunizations and other preventive care, and the hospital had a clear responsibility to assure that satisfactory arrangements were made, parents understood the arrangements, and recommended services were received.

Prior to the development of GHS, arrangements for the care of staff-delivered infants were coordinated by the Outpatient Department. A nurse or pediatric house officer contacted the mother before her discharge from the hospital and scheduled an appointment for the well-baby clinic, unless the mother indicated that she planned to take the baby elsewhere for care. A home visit by a public health nurse routinely was made soon after, and a second visit was made if the clinic appointment was not kept. At six to twelve months of age, the child was referred to the pediatric clinic for further care.

Currently, after delivery by a GHS obstetrician, each baby is examined by a GHS pediatrician, who also talks with the mother prior to discharge. Arrangements are made for a GHS appointment in about three weeks, unless the mother indicates other plans. If the initial appointment is not kept, the physician supervises follow-up by a nurse practitioner, nurse, or secretary. Only if special circumstances warrant is a home visit by a public-health nurse arranged.

Methods. The study was designed to make two types of comparisons between the services received from the pediatric clinics and those received from GHS: the relative success in bringing the staff-delivered infants into the ambulatory-care program, and, for those children seen in the program, the relative adequacy of the timing and completion of recognized preventive procedures. Two samples of staff-attended pregnancies were selected from the hospital's inpatient registry. The first sample ($n = 100$) was chosen from a universe of 499 births that occurred in the period October 1969–September 1970; the second sample, of equal size, from 333 births between June 1973 and May 1974. Care subsequently received in OPD by newborns from the first sample prior to May 30, 1971 was abstracted from hospital medical records. GHS charts were used to document the care received by the second sample prior to February 28, 1975. All children in both samples were between nine and twenty-one months of age at the end of the study periods. The study periods were chosen to provide the most recent data available at the time of the sampling in March 1975, while isolating clinic services from the effects of GHS planning and organizational change.

For each case in which an initial visit had been made, we examined the charts to determine whether a set of immunizations and screening procedures had been completed. A child for whom a given preventive procedure had not been completed was considered behind schedule if his age exceeded by more than two months the recommended age for completion. We also documented acute visits, emergency-room visits, and available sociodemographic information.

Results. Table 5–10 presents the sociodemographic characteristics of the two samples of newborns. The data confirm the high-risk nature of these target populations. The two samples are essentially similar, with one excep-

Table 5-10
Newborn Sample Characteristics

	OPD (N = 100)	GHS (N = 100)	p Value
A. Race/ethnicity (%)			
1. White	53	47	
2. Black	38	47	.38[a]
3. Spanish-surnamed	9	6	
B. Source of payment (%)			
1. Medicaid	75	72	
2. Other third party	16	20	.75[a]
3. No third party	9	9	
C. Parental circumstances (%)			
1. Mother living with spouse	46	41	
2. Other	54	59	.57[a]
D. Mother's age (mean year)	22.7	23.2	.52[b]
E. Duration of prenatal care (mean month)	3.6	4.6	.00[b]

Source: Ralph Ullman, David Kotok, and James R. Tobin, "Hospital-Based Group Practice and Comprehensive Care for Children of Indigent Families," *Pediatrics* 60 (1977): 873. Used with permission.

[a]Chi-square for difference in proportions, two-tailed.

[b]Student's *t* for difference in means, two-tailed.

tion—in the most recent period, the mothers tended to present earlier for prenatal care.

Table 5–11, part A, shows that plans for pediatric care at Genesee Hospital were made for relatively fewer of the earlier sample, primarily because of the large group of newborns who were placed for adoption. New York State's liberalized abortion legislation of 1971 probably was a factor in this remarkable difference between the two samples. Further, an increased tendency among unwed mothers to keep their babies was observed generally in the Rochester area.

The great majority of both groups of children for whom continued care at Genesee had been planned were brought in for at least one well-child visit (table 5–11, part B). However, the GHS "capture rate" of 97 percent is significantly greater than the 84 percent recorded for OPD. Among the children seen, clinic patients were three times as likely to be transferred later to another physician or health center (table 5–11, part C).

We used two measures to summarize the preventive care rendered to children who made at least one well-child visit:

1. The percentage of patients who were up to date on all procedures through the end of the study period (or, if a patient was transferred elsewhere, through the date of the last visit)
2. The percentage on schedule at least through the date of the last visit.

Table 5-11
Well-Baby Referral and Utilization

	OPD		GHS	
A. Well-baby referral				
1. OPD-GHS	75		91	
2. Other clinic/physician	8		5	
3. Adoption	15		0	
4. Perinatal mortality	2		3	
5. Nonobstetric maternal mortality	0		1	
Total	100		100	
B. For OPD-GHS referrals				
(line 1 of A): Well-baby visit made?				
1. Yes	63	(84%)	88	(97%)
2. No	12	(16%)	3	(3%)[a]
Total	75	(100%)	91	(100%)
C. For well-baby visitors (line 1 of B):				
Later transferred to other clinic/				
physician?				
1. Yes	19	(30%)	8	(9%)
2. No	44	(70%)	80	(91%)[a]
Total	63	(100%)	88	(100%)

Source: Ralph Ullman, David Kotok, and James R. Tobin, "Hospital-Based Group Practice and Comprehensive Care for Children of Indigent Families," *Pediatrics* 60 (1977): 873. Used with permission.

[a]$p \leq .01$, Chi-square for difference in proportions, one-tailed.

As table 5-12 (parts A and B) shows, on both measures GHS was more successful in achieving the timed completion of overall preventive care. While some of the seven procedures used as standard criteria presented difficulty in obtaining a fair comparison, more detailed analysis revealed that higher percentages of the GHS newborns were up to date on *each* procedure.[9]

The pattern of acute care received by the children who made at least one well-child visit is shown in table 5-12, parts C and D. The data are consistent with what we have observed for the pediatric practice as a whole. The GHS newborns were more likely to have been seen for an acute visit in the same facility and less likely to have been taken to the emergency room.

Several cautions should be exercised when interpreting the comparative results of this study. First, since OPD and GHS records were unlikely to document care rendered by other sources, the derived immunization and utilization rates are only lower bounds for the total care received. Second, contributions to the improved screening and immunization status of Genesee-born infants may have resulted from the abortion legislation, changed social values, or other community-wide phenomena. However, confirmatory evidence of the effectiveness of the pediatric group in providing care to children of indigent families has been documented by other researchers.[10] They found GHS to compare favorably with two community health centers in:

1. Completion of immunizations for children of teen-aged mothers
2. Resolution of anemia in infants
3. Lowered morbidity of children with bronchial asthma.

We conclude from these and our earlier data on utilization that low-income families have been integrated successfully into the GHS pediatric practice.

A Redistribution of Resources

The sociodemographic comparisons of the present chapter, together with the information on the growth of the Genesee Health Service presented in chapter 4, demonstrate convincingly that the program has effected an increased utilization of primary-care services at the hospital by low-income, inner-city residents. Yet, as this trend became evident to us, we had to remind ourselves that, from a broader social perspective, GHS did not represent a new and otherwise unavailable resource. Had the new group not been formed, all of the physicians would have been providing medical care in one setting or another. We debated, therefore, whether GHS had functioned truly as a mechanism for the redistribution of medical resources toward

Table 5-12
Services Received by Well-Baby Visitors

	OPD		*GHS*	
A. Preventive care up to date through end of study period?				
1. Yes	25	(40%)	58	(66%)
2. No	38	(60%)	30	(34%)[a]
B. Preventive care up to date through date of last visit?				
1. Yes	45	(71%)	81	(92%)
2. No	18	(29%)	7	(8%)[a]
C. OPD-GHS acute visits				
1. None	42	(67%)	22	(25%)
2. One or more	21	(33%)	66	(75%)[a]
D. Genesee ED visits				
1. None	18	(29%)	49	(56%)
2. One or more	45	(71%)	39	(44%)[a]
Total	63	(100%)	88	(100%)

Source: Ralph Ullman, David Kotok, and James R. Tobin, "Hospital-Based Group Practice and Comprehensive Care for Children of Indigent Families," *Pediatrics* 60 (1977): 873. Used with permission.

Note: Cases in this table are those of line 1 of table 5-11, part B.

[a]$p \leq .01$, Chi-square for difference in proportions, one-tailed.

those who needed them the most. What were the motivations of the physicians in joining the practice, and what would they have been doing in its absence?

We reviewed a series of interviews conducted with thirteen GHS physicians, each relatively soon after initial employment.[11] The physicians expressed a variety of reasons for joining GHS, which were categorized as either "organizationally related" or "patient-related" factors. All physicians mentioned at least one organizationally related factor, such as financial viability, convenience to hospital facilities, guaranteed first-year salary, opportunity to participate in teaching and professional activities, attractiveness of a medium-sized group practice, sharing night and weekend coverage, and freedom from administrative details.

Patient-related factors concerning the attractiveness of the anticipated GHS patient population were mentioned by six physicians as a reason for joining the practice. For three of these physicians, patient-related factors appeared to be dominant; for the other three, organizationally related factors were more important.

In summary, as GHS planners had anticipated, the establishment of a program designed specifically to treat a broad cross-section of the community did seem to have been an important positive factor in physician recruitment. Clearly this factor did not dominate other characteristics of the program. It appears that some physicians already were oriented toward group practice, and that they made their choices primarily on the basis of comparative advantages in convenience, location, and professional advancement. Other physicians expressed more interest in the patients they would be treating, and in the resultant effect on themselves as practitioners. It does seem unlikely that the majority of the GHS physicians interviewed would have accepted employment in a program directed solely at a poverty population. Therefore, with respect to increasing the availability of personal physicians among the poor, the Genesee Health Service must be regarded as a success.

Financial Impact and the Cost of Care

From the viewpoint of Genesee Hospital administrators, the reorganization of outpatient services initially appeared to present several financial advantages. First, the grants for construction of the Genesee Health Service facility enabled an immediate increase in the value of the hospital's physical plant. Second, the anticipated increase in the size of the middle-class segment of the outpatient population could lead to greater use and reimbursement of profitable ancillary services and could provide a larger group of patients who might require hospitalization. Third, OEO's promise of deficit financing for the first several years of GHS operation assured at least a short-term improvement in the hospital's financial position, since OPD customarily incurred a net loss. Finally, administrators hoped that by the time federal funding was no longer available, tightened fiscal management would enable long-term operation of GHS on a break-even basis, or at least with less of an annual deficit than had characterized OPD.

The duration of our research project was a very short period within which to assess the financial impact of the reorganization on the sponsoring institution. We decided to attempt this assessment, however, primarily in order to gain a perspective on the longer-term fiscal prospects of GHS. Moreover, we wished to examine the impact of the program on the cost of providing care.[12]

Our general strategy required, first, that we prepare an income statement for OPD's activities in 1971, its last full year of operation, and, then, that we compare these data with a similar statement prepared for GHS in 1974, the most recent year for which complete data were available. These statements could be compared only with respect to the outpatient facilities, to the exclusion of ancillary and inpatient services. Supplemental to the income statements were the total costs of providing service, which were computed by adding to the hospital's expenses any costs of physician time not borne by the hospital. Division of these costs by the appropriate numbers of visits yielded cost-per-visit ratios with respect to which OPD and GHS can be compared also.

Our calculations showed a net loss of approximately $70,000 attributable to the operation of the entire OPD in 1971. Although the allocations of revenues and expenses did not necessarily conform to the hospital's standard accounting procedures, this figure was within the range of estimates previously made by the administration regarding the annual loss. Our analysis showed, however, that only about $30,000 of the deficit could be attributed to the clinics that GHS replaced. The remainder was associated with other clinics and ancillary services.

Our construction of a GHS financial statement for 1974 demonstrated a sizable operating deficit of about $235,000. Some portion of this deficit was attributable to costs of providing care being greater than the fees charged to patients, some attributable to a substantial problem in collection of fees charged, and some (perhaps $60,000) to unreimbursed expenses of administrating the OEO grant. Since the grant fully covered all operating deficits, the hospital incurred no net loss related to GHS and thereby gained a modest financial benefit from its reorganization of outpatient services. Based on a strict comparison between OPD and GHS, $30,000 is a realistic estimate of the annual savings accrued through the deficit financing of the federal grant. The GHS income statement, however, showed that, albeit in a period of rapid growth, the fiscal self-sufficiency of the program was not imminent. While the medical group probably was strong enough to become independent of the federal subsidy, it seems clear also that such action would have affected seriously their ability to attain their objectives, in particular, the provision of care to patients with inadequate financial resources. It has been observed that the reform of ambulatory-care delivery nationally has been constrained severely by the country's pattern of health financing.[13] We know of no more recent information that would be reason to change this basic conclusion.

Table 5-13 presents the OPD and GHS cost-per-visit ratios, which were $12.91 and $20.50, respectively, averaged over all the primary-care specialties. Viewed on this basis, GHS medical care was 59 percent more costly than comparable services rendered by OPD three years earlier. Most of the increase was due to a major change in physician staffing. The GHS medical group is composed predominantly of full-time, board-certified specialists. OPD depended heavily on the part-time availability of much lower-salaried house officers of the hospital. We argue previously that GHS did not constitute an otherwise unavailable resource; similarly, we argue now that a redistribution of physician effort per se did not change the total cost to the community. Accordingly, if we control for the difference between OPD and GHS in physician cost per visit, there remains only a 19 percent increase to be explained by other factors. The figure is not much higher than the 16 percent inflation experienced by the national Medical Care Price Index between mid-1971 and mid-1974. Thus, the rise in the cost of a primary-care visit does not appear excessive when placed against the changed nature of the service itself. We leave the final judgment, of course, to the reader.

Table 5-13
OPD-GHS Cost Comparison

	(1971) OPD	(1974) GHS
Direct	$ 85,424	
Indirect from hospital—physicians	21,145	
Other indirect expenses	77,266	
Physicians		$382,074
Supporting personnel		372,876
Other operating expenses		213,307
Total expenses	$183,835	$968,257
Cost of additional physicians' time	$ 32,000	$ 15,559
Total costs	$215,835	$981,608
Visits	16,717	47,883
Cost per visit	$12.91	$20.50

Notes

1. George S. Paxton, John A. Sbarbaro, and Nicholas Mossaman, "A Core City Problem: Recruitment and Retention of Salaried Physicians," *Medical Care* 13(1975):209.

2. Margaret C. Heagarty and Leon S. Robertson, "Slave Doctors and Free Doctors: A Participant Observer Study of the Physician-Patient Relationship in a Low-Income Comprehensive-Care Program." *New England Journal of Medicine* 284(1971):636.

3. Ralph Ullman, "A Report of Telephone Utilization at the Genesee Health Service," mimeographed (Rochester, N.Y.: Health Services Research Center, The Genesee Hospital, 1975).

4. Louis I. Hochheiser, Kenneth Woodward, and Evan Charney, "Effect of the Neighborhood Health Center on the Use of Pediatric Emergency Departments in Rochester, New York," *New England Journal of Medicine* 285(1971):148; Gordon T. Moore, Roberta Bernstein, and Rosemary A. Bonanno, "Effect of a Neighborhood Health Center on Hospital Emergency Room Use," *Medical Care* 10(1972):240; Klaus J. Roghmann and Hyman J.V. Goldberg, "Effect of Rochester Neighborhood Health Center on Hospital Dental Emergencies," *Medical Care* 12(1974):251.

5. The last analysis has been reported previously as Ralph Ullman et al., "Impact of a Primary Care Group Practice on Emergency Room Utilization at a Community Hospital," *Medical Care* 16(1978):723.

6. Hochheiser, Woodward, and Charney, "Effect of the Neighborhood Health Center."

7. Eugene Vayda, Michael Gent, and Linda Paisley, "An Emergency Department Triage Model Based on Presenting Complaints," *Canadian Journal of Public Health* 64(1973):246.

8. This section is adapted from an article that appeared previously as Ralph Ullman, David Kotok, and James R. Tobin, "Hospital-Based Group Practice and Comprehensive Care for Children of Indigent Families," *Pediatrics* 60(1977):873. Used with permission.

9. Ibid., table IV, p. 878.

10. Owen Mathieu et al., "Does Team Organization and Outreach Effect Outcome? A Comparison of Three Neighborhood Health Centers," abstracted, *Pediatric Research* 10(1976):306.

11. Ralph Ullman, "The Practicing Physician and the 'One-Class' System of Care," mimeographed (Rochester, N.Y.: Health Services Research Center, The Genesee Hospital, 1975). The cited interviews were conducted by Donna I. Regenstreif, who provided the authors the responses relevant to the issues addressed here. The identities of individual respondents were not disclosed. See also Donna I. Regenstreif, "Innovation in Hospital-Based Ambulatory Care: Some Sources, Patterns and Implications of Change," *Human Organization* 36(1977):43.

12. Ralph Ullman, "A Financial Analysis Relating to the Development of the Genesee Health Service," mimeographed (Rochester, N.Y.: Health Services Research Center, The Genesee Hospital, 1975).

13. Robert J. Blendon, "The Reform of Ambulatory Care: A Financial Paradox," *Medical Care* 14(1976):526.

6 Patients' Perceptions

In chapter 2 we describe in detail a study of community attitudes about ambulatory-care delivery. Our purpose in that study was primarily to establish the criteria that people use to judge health-care delivery in the ambulatory setting. While the findings were of general interest, the application of the model of rational patient behavior was undertaken with the later intent of comparing these community attitudes to those of Genesee Health Service patients. We wanted to determine whether planners were correct in their view of what they thought patients expected from an ambulatory-care service. As important, we wanted to determine how patients evaluated the new health service with respect to these evaluative components. If planners were correct in their intuitive understanding of what patients expected, and if the new service met those expectations, it should be relatively easy to elicit patient opinions on this subject. And, such a survey also would permit comparative analysis of services rendered within GHS. For example, the information about utilization and impact that we discuss in the previous chapter suggests somewhat greater effectiveness of the pediatric practice in achieving goals of rapport, compliance, and so forth. One would expect that these findings might be reinforced with more positive expressions of patient satisfaction toward the pediatric practice than for the other specialties. From the perspective of our overall evaluation, the study of patient satisfaction was therefore an important complement to the studies of impact and utilization.

Our conduct of the patient satisfaction study proved more difficult than we had anticipated. We encountered a profound problem, one that we believe has important implications for other research in which the strategy involves at-home interviews with an inner-city population of respondents. We discuss first this confounding issue because of its obvious relevance to our findings about how GHS patients assessed the new health-care program.

Material in this chapter has been adapted from William C. Stratmann, "A Group Medical Practice Replaces a Hospital's Outpatient Clinics: An Appraisal of Patient Satisfaction," mimeographed (Rochester, N.Y.: Health Services Research Center, The Genesee Hospital, 1975).

Sampling Procedure

Between the inception of GHS in early 1972 and October 1974, the specialties of pediatrics, internal medicine, and obsterics/gynecology treated approximately fifteen thousand patients. For the empirical study of utilization, our sample consisted of every fifteenth medical record. For practical reasons, we chose to use this same sample as a population base for the patient survey. To create an appropriate subsample for the survey from this representative base, we first excluded all ob/gyn records, because we believed that insufficient time had elapsed for this practice to become stabilized. Thus we decided to focus only on the pediatric and medical specialties, which produced an initial sample of 884 patient names, about equally divided between the two groups. Practical reasons and the purpose of the survey dictated further reduction of the sample. Our primary populations of interest were patients in medicine and the parents of pediatric patients whom we could assume had used GHS as their primary source of care and who could report their views of the new service without difficulty to a professional staff of interviewers. Budgetary concerns also necessitated that we limit the travel of interviewers so far as was practical. Accordingly, we eliminated from the sample patients (or parents of patients) who:

1. Were less than seventeen years old, were senile, or had language problems or a speaking disability,
2. Resided more than fifteen miles from the GHS facility,
3. Had not visited GHS subsequent to March 1973, when the practice moved into its permanent office space, or
4. Had made fewer than two visits.

These operational and study constraints reduced the original pediatric/medical sample to 516 prospective respondents.

To each of the remaining sampled individuals, we addressed letters, using the most recent address in their medical records, inviting their participation in the survey. An initial letter was sent by the GHS Medical Director:

Dear _____
You probably know that, as a hospital-based group medical practice, the Genesee Health Service is a relatively new approach to health care delivery. So new, in fact, that the Genesee Hospital has received a grant to support a study of the Genesee Health Service. The study will try to find out whether the people who have used the Health Service think we are meeting our goal of trying to provide better health care to those in need of medical help.

I am writing to invite you to participate in a survey of Genesee Health Service patients. The names of the people whom we would like to interview have been picked at random from among 15,000 patients who have used the Health Service. Your name is one of those that were chosen by chance.

The purpose of the survey is to find out what patients think about the Genesee Health Service — the office, staff, and so forth. Your answers to the interviewer's questions will of course be held in confidence, you will not be asked any questions about your medical problems or the medical treatment you've received, and you will not be identified in any report that evolves from the study.

If you would prefer not to participate in the survey please phone my secretary at _____, and inform her that you do not wish to be interviewed. If we don't hear from you within a week I will assume that you are willing to participate in the survey.

Sincerely,

Medical Director

We had several concerns that prompted our wording in the letters that invited respondent participation. First, we did not wish to impose on any patient or parent. Indeed, this was a concern also of members of the Health Service Board, who approved of our strategy and who, incidentally, participated in a pretest of the eventual survey protocol so as to assure themselves of the innocuous nature of the study. As important, however, was our awareness of the potential difficulty we might have in convincing people to permit themselves to be interviewed. We therefore wrote an additional letter, this time over the signature of the research director:

Dear _____
A week ago Dr. _____, Medical Director of the Genesee Health Service, invited you to participate in our research study. The purpose of the study is to determine how parents feel about the health services their children receive.

We have designed a questionaire that will be administered by _____, a locally based professional survey organization. A representative of this organization will contact you in a week or so to make an appointment for a personal interview.

If you would prefer not to participate in our study please call my secretary, _____, phone _____, and she will remove your name from our list. I should mention, however, that I think you will enjoy our interview. Our experience has been that people get pleasure from an opportunity to offer their opinion of health services.

Unless I hear otherwise I will assume that a representative of _____, may telephone you to make an appointment for an interview.

May I express my appreciation in advance for your cooperation. Only with the help of those who use health care facilities can we determine our progress toward the goal of providing for the kind of health care services they want.

Sincerely,

Research Director

Addressees of the first letter who took the action of requesting that their names be deleted from our list were not sent the second letter. We received a total of only twenty-one requests for nonparticipation. Our initial feeling of elation at having so many willing respondents was short-lived. The basic sample of 516 was reduced further because many people simply could not be located. Fifty-eight letters were returned marked "no such number," twenty-seven were returned marked "left no forwarding address," and twenty were returned marked "address unknown." It was obvious that we had a problem. We were astounded at the apparent mobility of these patients, who for the most part lived in the inner city. Our problem became larger after we gave the remaining 373 names, addresses, and telephone numbers to the professional research organization. Fifty-nine people on the list flatly refused to be interviewed. A surprising 101 additional people could not be located, either by telephone or as a result of several attempts to locate the respondent at his residence. In some instances, interviewers tracked prospective respondents to two or three different addresses before admitting defeat in not being able to locate an individual. Not infrequently, interviewers reported their belief that a respondent was home but refused to answer the door. In sum, notwithstanding what we believed was a nonthreatening approach to our sample of respondents, and notwithstanding the very diligent efforts of the interviewers, we were able to complete interviews with only 119 adult patients and the parents (usually the mothers) of 105 pediatric patients.

The great majority of the patients whom we could not interview were inner-city residents. Our interviewers reported that among this population there was a strong distrust of strangers. Interviewers believed that some respondents viewed the survey as a subterfuge, suspecting the interviewer to be a bill collector. Others apparently desired simply to remain anonymous. For whatever reason, the problem that we encountered has obvious implications for any form of attitudinal research that is dependent on the cooperation of a population of specific service users.

The reliability and validity of our findings are a function of the representativeness of our sample. To what extent our findings are biased by the poor response rate we can only speculate. One can argue that patients who chose not to be interviewed were more likely to be those who were dissatisfied with the new service. Conversely, one might expect the dissatisfied segment to be more, rather than less motivated to take advantage of a forum that enabled them to voice their discontent.

Our questionnaire was lengthy, and we did not wish to impose on patient, provider, or staff by holding extensive interviews in the office setting. Further, we believe that the patient's home is the most suitable place to obtain objective responses. We suspect that our missing respondents were little more likely to be either satisfied or dissatisified with GHS than were those of similar sociodemographic background who were interviewed, in part because the findings of the survey seem consistent with the earlier data on utilization and impact. But we frankly are perplexed by the nonresponse problem and at a loss to suggest how one might achieve a higher response rate under similar circumstances.

The Patient Survey

The survey protocol was patterned after the instrument used in the survey of the Rochester community. Open-ended questions were used to elicit from patients the factors that influenced their decision to use the Genesee Health Service as a source of ambulatory care. The respondent later was asked to rank-order these decision-components, as in the community survey, and to assign to them measures of importance using a ten-point scale. Then the respondent was asked to indicate his satisfaction with sources previously or since utilized, with respect to each of the decision-components. The decision-components were categorized and compared with the opinions expressed by the Rochester community. The satisfaction values also were combined to give overall ratings of different sources that the respondent had used. In addition to the open-ended approach, respondents were asked a series of close-ended questions about the process of care. The questions were based on information about patient concerns obtained from the community survey. With respect to each specific aspect of the care process, current GHS patients were asked to compare the new program with the source of care previously used most often. Respondents who no longer used GHS were asked to compare it with the facility then used most often.

While the primary purpose of the survey was to elicit patient satisfaction with the Genesee Health Service, other areas of interest were investigated also. In awareness of the goal of gaining patient reliance on GHS for care, even in emergencies, respondents were asked what they would do for after-hour needs. We also desired to determine respondent attitudes toward such things as the use of physician assistants, prepayment plans, and incidents that may have angered or annoyed them. The usual sociodemographic data were obtained so as to develop a profile of the respondent population.

Sociodemographic Comparisons

Table 6-1 compares the respondent sample with the representative utilization sample on the basis of race and source of payment. As we can infer from our difficulties in completing interviews in the inner city, the respondents in both specialty groups underrepresent the proportion of Medicaid patients in the GHS population. Correspondingly, black patients also are underrepresented in the surveyed sample of patients in medicine, although apparently not so in the pediatric sample. Table 6-2 presents a broader sociodemographic profile of the respondent samples and also furnishes a comparison with the community survey described in chapter 2.

Previously Used Sources of Care

Hospital outpatient departments and private doctors were the sources of care most frequently used by the respondents before coming to the Genesee Health Service (see table 6-3). Of those who used hospital clinics, the majority were former Genesee clinic patients, as expected. A significant proportion of the respondents, however, were attracted from other hospital outpatient clinics in the Rochester area. Although a smaller number of respondents were habitual users of emergency rooms, for both pediatrics

Table 6-1
Sociodemographics of Survey and Utilization Samples

| | Patient Type | | | |
| | Pediatrics | | Medicine | |
Characteristics	(1) Survey Sample	(2) Utilization Sample	(1) Survey Sample	(2) Utilization Sample
Race				
White	61	59	76	64
Black	37	37	23	32
Spanish-speaking	2	4	2	4
Source of payment				
Medicaid	26	46	10	32
Non-Medicaid	74	54	90	68

Table 6-2
Sociodemographic Characteristics of Survey Respondents
(percent)

Characteristics	(1) Pediatric Patients	(2) Medical Patients	(3) Community Survey
Race			
Black	37	23	10
White	61	76	90
Spanish	2	2	1
Sex			
Male	3	41	40
Female	97	59	60
Income			
< $2,500	11	13	2
2,500-4,999	14	17	6
5,000-7,499	10	10	8
7,500-9,999	11	7	9
10,000-12,499	19	10	17
12,500-14,999	9	7	13
15,000-19,999	9	12	20
≥ 20,000	7	15	15
Don't know/refused	11	9	12
Employment			
Employed full-time	29	48	33
Employed part-time	14	8	10
Retired	1	14	14
Unemployed	11	17	3
Full-time student	0	3	1
Housewife	46	11	38
Marital status			
Married—living with spouse	54	45	81
Separated	17	11	2
Divorced	13	7	3
Widow/widower	2	13	8
Single	11	19	7
Single—common-law spouse	2	3	0
Religion			
Protestant	51	45	44
Catholic	30	32	46
Jewish	0	2	2
Other	18	20	5
No Answer	0	2	2
Education			
≤ 8 grade	9	17	12
> 8, ≥ 12 grade	67	46	48
> 12 grade	25	37	40
Age			
17-25	24	13	11
26-35	54	26	26
36-45	14	20	17
46-55	6	13	18
56-65	1	18	13
> 65	0	10	14

Table 6-2 (continued)

Characteristics	(1) Pediatric Patients	(2) Medical Patients	(3) Community Survey
Insurance coverage			
None	5	16	3
Blue Cross/Blue Shield	51	37	73
Medicare	5	10	2
Medicaid	26	10	5
Other	14	28	18

and medicine about half of these came from hospitals other than Genesee. Medical patients, in the main, reported private practices as former sources of care. Only a few medical patients indicated no former source. The relatively larger number of pediatric respondents in this category is misleading, since they consist primarily of parents whose first source of care for a newborn infant was GHS. At the time of the survey, about 9 percent of the combined sample (seven parents and twelve medical patients) had decided to discontinue use of GHS in favor of another source of care. Their new sources varied widely. We learned from analysis of patient records that 74 percent of the pediatric sample and 83 percent of the medical sample had utilized GHS in the previous twelve months.

Relative Importance of Decision-Components

In the study of community attitudes about health care, we collapsed reported decision-components into five categories: economic, temporal, convenience, sociopsychological, and quality factors. In our earlier discussion of these factors, we note that perceptions of the relative importance of these criterion categories do not correlate closely with sociodemographic characteristics. Table 6-4 presents criteria weightings by sex for both the GHS patient survey and the community survey. It is apparent that the women in the GHS medical sample, who sought care for themselves, differed in their opinions about the relative importance of decision-components from the women interviewed in the pediatric sample. Convenience, in particular, was more important to respondents in the pediatric sample. Among medical respondents, the attitudes of males differed only slightly from those of females.

Attitudes of adult GHS respondents differed from their counterparts in the community. Temporal and convenience factors were less important to the GHS samples than to the community as a whole. Correspondingly, sociopsychological factors were quite a bit more important. This finding

Table 6-3
Previously Used Sources of Care for GHS Patients

	Patient Sample			
	Pediatrics		Medicine	
Source	%	(N)	%	(N)
Hospital clinic				
Genesee Hospital	21	(20)	17	(18)
Other	14	(13)	8	(8)
Total	35	(33)	25	(26)
Hospital emergency room				
Genesee	4	(4)	3	(3)
Other	4	(4)	4	(4)
Total	8	(8)	7	(7)
Private doctor				
Single practice	34	(32)	55	(58)
Group practice	4	(4)	3	(3)
Total	38	(36)	58	(61)
Neighborhood health center	6	(6)	5	(5)
Clinic at work	—	—	3	(3)
VA clinic	—	—	1	(1)
Other	1	(1)	—	—
None	12	(11)	2	(2)
Total	100	(95)	101	(105)

supports the belief of those who planned the new service that care to the target population should be delivered in a setting and manner that befits the dignity and privacy of each patient, and that a mutually satisfying personal relationship should be established between the patient and the physician. Table 6-5 affords a comparison of the sample of GHS patients with respondents in the community survey who customarily used other sources of care. The attitudes of GHS patients

Table 6-4
Relative Importance of Decision-Components

	Criterion						
Sample Characteristic	Economic	Temporal	Convenience	Sociopsychological	Quality		N
	(%)	(%)	(%)	(%)	(%)	(%)	No.
GHS							
Male patient	4.3	7.6	13.3	34.4	40.4	100	(49)
Female patient	5.6	4.7	12.7	31.5	45.4	100	(70)
Female parent	3.5	9.7	20.4	24.8	41.6	100	(102)
Population Survey							
Male	4.8	12.0	22.6	15.8	44.7	100	(187)
Female	3.2	11.0	18.1	23.5	44.0	100	(323)

Table 6-5
Criterion Importance by Facility Used Most Often

| Facility Used Most Often | Criterion | | | | | N | |
	Economic (%)	Temporal (%)	Convenience (%)	Sociopsychological (%)	Quality (%)	(%)	No
Hospital emergency room	7.0	11.4	29.2	9.9	41.8	100	(7
Hospital clinic	7.2	14.1	12.7	20.8	45.2	100	(40
Private physician	2.6	11.4	20.2	20.5	45.3	100	(320
Clinic at work	7.7	13.0	19.0	16.1	44.2	100	(20
Neighborhood health center	8.4	9.5	10.6	27.2	44.3	100	(15
Genesee Health Service	4.3	7.5	16.1	29.1	42.6	100	(224

toward the relative importance of criteria categories most closely resemble those of people in the community survey who used neighborhood health centers.

Comparative Measures of Patient Satisfaction

Two different questioning techniques were used to derive comparative measures of patient satisfaction. Both techniques required the respondent to compare the Genesee Health Service with another source of care, that now used, or that previously used by the respondent, with respect to specific factors that we had derived from our study of community standards for health-care delivery. Table 6-6 illustrates the first technique—

Table 6-6
Comparative Satisfaction of GHS Patients with Previous Source of Care

Category		Pediatrics %	Medicine %
1. "Is the location of the GHS more convenient, about the same, or less convenient?"	More Convenient	41	42
	About the Same	37	42
	Less Convenient	22	15
	Don't Know	—	1
2. "Does the GHS cost more, about the same, or less?"	Costs More	15	26
	About the Same	44	26
	Costs Less	23	21
	Don't Know	17	26
3. "At the GHS do you spend more, about the same, or less time waiting?"	More Time	7	10
	About the Same	15	28
	Less Time	78	62
	Don't Know	—	1
4. "Do the people at the GHS treat you as a person better, about the same, or worse?"	Better	48	40
	About the Same	50	57
	Worse	2	2
	Don't Know	—	1

Table 6-6 (continued)

Category		Pediatrics %	Medicine %
5. "Is the quality of medical care better, about the same, or worse?"	Better	61	54
	About the Same	37	39
	Worse	1	2
	Don't Know	1	5
6. "As far as physical comfort, is the GHS more comfortable, about the same, or less comfortable?"	More Comfortable	80	64
	About the Same	19	31
	Less Comfortable	1	2
	Don't Know	—	3
7. "When you walk into the GHS do you feel more at ease, about the same, or less at ease?"	More at Ease	73	56
	About the Same	24	35
	Less at Ease	2	6
	Don't Know	—	3
8. "Are the GHS office hours more convenient, about the same, or less convenient?"	More Convenient	69	48
	About the Same	24	41
	Less Convenient	2	6
	Don't Know	5	6
9. "At the GHS, do you see the same doctor more often, about the same, or less often?"	More Often	65	45
	About the Same	22	43
	Less Often	8	4
	Don't Know	5	9
10. "At the GHS, are the doctors more friendly, about the same, or less friendly?"	More Friendly	59	38
	About the Same	37	55
	Less Friendly	2	5
	Don't Know	1	2
11. "At the GHS, do you think the doctors care more, about the same, or less?"	Care More	61	42
	About the Same	34	49
	Care Less	2	6
	Don't Know	4	4
12. "At the GHS, do you think the doctors are more experienced, about the same, or less experienced?"	More Experienced	42	31
	About the Same	47	39
	Less Experienced	6	16
	Don't Know	6	13
13. "At the GHS, do you think the nurses and staff care more, about the same, or care less?"	Care More	64	42
	About the Same	35	47
	Care Less	1	8
	Don't Know	—	4
14. "At the GHS, are the doctors older, about the same age, or younger?"	Older	9	11
	About the Same	44	30
	Younger	38	54
	Don't Know	8	6
15. "Considering everything, convenience, cost, quality of care, and so on, are you more satisfied, or less satisfied than you were where you used to go for care?"	More Satisfied	81	68
	About the Same	14	29
	Less Satisfied	5	2
	Don't Know	—	1

patient perceptions of GHS respective to previous sources of care. The satisfaction of GHS respondents was broad-based, with parents of children who used the service generally more satisfied than medical patients. In table 6-7, we employ the same evaluative criteria while controlling for patient's

Table 6-7
Relationship between Previous Source of Care and
Comparative Satisfaction
(*percent*)

| | Previous Source of Care | | | | | |
| | Pediatrics | | | Medicine | | |
Category	Private	Clinic	Other	Private	Clinic	Other
Convenience						
More	40	37	45	48	16	50
Same	26	63	36	38	79	25
Less	34	0	21	15	5	25
	100%	100%	100%	101%[a]	100%	100%
Cost						
More	16	19	21	35	56	29
Same	45	56	63	29	33	59
Less	39	25	17	37	11	12
	100%	100%	101%	100%	100%	100%
Waiting Time						
More	8	0	10	15	5	0
Same	29	5	3	36	16	17
Less	63	95	86	49	79	83
	100%	100%	99%	100%	100%	100%
Personal Treatment						
Better	32	79	48	34	32	63
Same	63	21	52	62	68	38
Worse	5	0	0	3	0	0
	100%	100%	100%	99%	100%	101%
Quality of Care						
Better	46	79	69	53	63	61
Same	54	21	28	45	37	35
Worse	0	0	3	2	0	4
	100%	100%	100%	101%	100%	100%
Physical Comfort						
Better	68	100	83	52	90	83
Same	29	0	17	45	11	17
Worse	3	0	0	3	0	0
	100%	100%	100%	100%	101%	100%
Ease of Feeling						
More	53	100	83	40	74	91
Same	42	0	17	53	21	4
Less	5	0	0	7	5	4
	100%	100%	100%	100%	100%	99%

Table 6-7 (continued)

| | Previous Source of Care | | | | | |
| | Pediatrics | | | Medicine | | |
Category	Private	Clinic	Other	Private	Clinic	Other
Convenience of Office Hours						
More	61	95	70	48	74	38
Same	39	5	22	48	26	48
Less	0	0	7	5	0	14
	100%	100%	99%	101%	100%	100%
Same Doctor						
More Often	36	94	93	28	77	82
Equally	44	6	7	68	18	14
Less Often	19	0	0	4	5	5
	99%	100%	100%	100%	101%	101%
Friendliness of Doctors						
More	43	79	69	36	32	52
Same	51	21	31	56	68	48
Less	5	0	0	8	0	0
	99%	100%	100%	100%	100%	100%
Concern of Doctor						
More	44	83	72	37	63	44
Same	50	17	28	53	37	57
Less	6	0	0	10	0	0
	100%	100%	100%	100%	100%	100%
Experience of Doctor						
More	22	74	54	17	65	65
Same	64	26	46	56	29	30
Less	14	0	0	28	6	5
	100%	100%	100%	101%	100%	100%
Concern of Staff						
More	66	74	57	36	37	70
Same	34	26	43	54	58	26
Less	0	0	0	10	5	4
	100%	100%	100%	100%	100%	100%
General Satisfaction						
Greater	68	100	86	60	74	87
Same	24	0	10	37	26	13
Less	8	0	3	3	0	0
	100%	100%	99%	100%	100%	100%

[a]Some columns do not sum to 100% because of rounding.

previous source of care. The groupings of patients are designed to enable comparison of former Genesee clinic users with former private and other patients. The least differential in satisfaction between former and present sources was reported by patients who previously had used a private physician for care. This is not surprising, since GHS was designed to create the appearance of a private practice setting. Yet, even among this group of patients a significantly greater degree of satisfaction with GHS was expressed for all categories, with only 8 percent indicating that they were less satisfied with the new service. The greatest level of comparative satisfaction was expressed by former users of Genesee's pediatric clinics.

The second technique used to document comparative satisfaction we believe to be more objective than the first. The reader will recall our discussion in chapter 2 in which we argue that aggregate analysis of attitudinal data derived from conventional survey questions may be invalid because it involves interpersonal comparisons of utility. It was this methodological dilemma that led to our model of patient decision-making. By focusing on the decisional circumstance, in this case the patient's selection of a source of care, the derived evaluative parameters circumvent the problem of interpersonal utility comparison because they are grounded on a common basis for measurement. In chapter 2 we test our model by comparing the calculated rational choice of facility with that most frequently used. A simple algorithm is employed to calculate normalized scores for each alternative facility type, based on a maximum of 100 percent. We use similar data from the patient survey to calculate normalized values that reflect a respondent's overall assessment of both GHS and the previously used facility.

Table 6-8 presents the normalized assessments of satisfaction. The figures in roman type represent the assessment of the Genesee Health Service; figures in italics represent the assessment of the previous source of care. Generally, higher scores were derived respective to GHS. This is particularly true for patients who formerly used the Genesee outpatient clinics. Interestingly, in assessments of the *former* source of care, previous Genesee clinic users also rated that facility consistently higher than the other two categories of patients rated their former sources of care. Among former Genesee clinic patients, males rated the clinics higher than did females, whites lower than did blacks, and people with less educational background higher than did others. At face value one might assume the relatively high assessments of Genesee's clinics to be an indication of superior service. It should be noted, however, that the group of former outpatients had no choice in their discontinuance of the clinics. All had to find another facility when the clinics were closed. Since most were referred directly to GHS, this group of respondents probably were reasonably representative of all former Genesee clinic patients with respect to their manifested satisfaction with that source of care. This is not true of the group of "other" patients, who changed from their previous source voluntarily and who therefore were more likely to represent the less satisfied users. Thus, this group assigned relatively low ratings to their former sources of care. This argument may hold also with respect to patients who formerly used a private physician, but to a lesser extent.

No clearly discernable pattern emerges from table 6-8 with respect to

Table 6-8
Normalized Preferences of Patients for Present and Previous Sources of Care

	Pediatrics			Medicine		
Characteristics	Private % (n)	Clinic % (n)	Other % (n)	Private % (n)	Clinic % (n)	Other % (n)
Sex						
Male	100.0 (1)	100.0 (1)	—	90.4 (26)	99.8 (5)	89.0 (12)
	30.6	*37.8*	—	*70.8*	*75.0*	*54.4*
Female	88.0 (38)	94.2 (18)	89.0 (39)	88.0 (35)	91.0 (14)	92.1 (13)
	72.8	*64.1*	*48.0*	*72.2*	*69.3*	*64.4*
Race						
Black	90.1 (11)	94.1 (7)	86.7 (20)	87.8 (9)	93.6 (4)	90.6 (12)
	74.8	*64.3*	*49.3*	*72.5*	*75.8*	*58.8*
White	87.0 (27)	94.8 (12)	91.4 (19)	88.9 (50)	93.2 (15)	89.7 (13)
	71.8	*61.7*	*46.2*	*71.6*	*69.5*	*60.4*
Income						
< $5,000	96.7 (7)	99.3 (4)	88.4 (15)	87.4 (16)	97.4 (9)	92.0 (8)
	59.0	*76.7*	*47.9*	*76.2*	*71.4*	*64.1*
5–10,000	87.5 (6)	91.8 (6)	91.5 (8)	89.9 (9)	91.0 (3)	97.7 (5)
	71.4	*64.4*	*60.2*	*70.3*	*85.9*	*69.0*
10–15,000	91.7 (12)	95.7 (5)	89.8 (9)	92.5 (8)	87.2 (2)	82.0 (7)
	77.3	*56.1*	*48.5*	*69.3*	*83.3*	*55.4*
15–20,000	82.7 (6)	—	78.2 (2)	81.3 (8)	—	93.6 (2)
	67.7	—	*40.2*	*74.8*	—	*27.5*
> 20,000	79.7 (5)	—	—	91.3 (15)	77.2 (1)	100.0 (2)
	80.2	—	—	*63.5*	*78.3*	*57.9*
Education						
≤ 8 Grade	—	—	89.1 (8)	95.2 (5)	95.3 (8)	92.6 (5)
	—	—	*44.5*	*73.4*	*64.1*	*72.1*
> 8, ≤ 12 Grade	88.1 (22)	94.7 (17)	88.3 (26)	87.4 (29)	91.6 (8)	93.0 (10)
	75.2	*62.0*	*50.9*	*68.3*	*72.9*	*57.5*
> 12 Grade	87.9 (16)	93.1 (2)	92.4 (5)	89.3 (6)	92.4 (3)	87.2 (10)
	68.5	*68.3*	*41.1*	*73.9*	*83.1*	*56.5*
Age						
17–25	93.7 (5)	92.7 (4)	91.3 (12)	84.2 (7)	83.8 (4)	85.4 (3)
	76.8	*87.0*	*54.0*	*65.2*	*57.2*	*56.8*
26–35	89.6 (28)	96.1 (8)	84.7 (17)	89.3 (12)	94.2 (6)	85.9 (7)
	70.5	*55.7*	*53.0*	*72.4*	*75.0*	*56.5*
36–45	74.1 (4)	94.4 (5)	95.2 (5)	86.7 (13)	100.0 (1)	95.5 (6)
	74.9	*54.9*	*33.1*	*65.8*	*84.5*	*65.5*
46–55	71.1 (1)	92.1 (2)	93.0 (3)	88.4 (10)	99.8 (2)	97.1 (2)
	86.4	*61.6*	*49.9*	*73.8*	*33.8*	*49.9*
56–65	—	—	80.7 (1)	97.2 (10)	91.0 (3)	91.5 (7)
	—	—	*58.7*	*69.5*	*93.9*	*61.5*
≥ 65	—	—	—	87.3 (9)	99.5 (3)	—
	—	—	—	*83.9*	*77.7*	—

present satisfaction with the Genesee Health Service when we control for the sociodemographic characteristics of the pediatric population. For the medical population, however, males seemed more satisfied with GHS than were females, especially among former Genesee clinic patients, and older people generally seemed more satisfied than younger people. Among this group of former clinic users, the GHS pediatric practice was slightly better received than the medical practice, consistent with the findings shown in table 6-7. In sum, the rating system does seem to be a sensitive measure of patient attitude.

Patient Dissatisfaction

Patients occasionally experience situations that annoy or anger them. Respondents were asked whether they had personally experienced such a situation and, if so, to describe what had happened. Of our sample of parents 30 percent reported such an incident, as did 38 percent of the medical sample. Of these, one-third of the parents who were offended reported that the incident made them change to another source of care. Of the adults who reported an incident, two-thirds changed. Twenty patients, about evenly divided between the two samples, reported experiencing such an incident at GHS. While five medical patients left for this reason, only one parent did so. Half of the incidents involved physicians. This same finding, incidentally, emerged from the community survey. Curiously, not a single GHS respondent complained about waiting time, which is often cited as a source of patient dissatisfaction, so much so that we asked the respondents several questions on the subject.

Respondents were asked to estimate their average waiting time at the Genesee Health Service, and whether this period of waiting time seemed reasonable to them. Median reported waiting time for both pediatrics and medicine was about thirteen minutes. Ninety-one percent of the parents believed their wait was reasonable; 93 percent of the medical patients. Only 10 percent of the parents reported waiting more than thirty minutes; only 6 percent of the medical patients. Twenty-eight percent of the parents reported waits of ten minutes or less, as opposed to 42 percent of the medical sample. Interestingly, although the medical group reported better performance from GHS on this parameter, reference to tables 6-6 and 6-7 indicates that the pediatric group reported relatively greater improvement over their former source of care. Their views are reinforced by reported estimates of how long a waiting period they had endured at their previous source. Fifty-seven percent of the parents reported waiting more than thirty minutes; 38 percent more than an hour. Of the medical sample 44 percent reported waits of more than a half hour; and an equal proportion waited more than an hour. Thus, the respondents' views on waiting time are consistent with the earlier data. The conventional perception of patient views on waiting time also was substantiated. Of the parents 54 percent thought the wait at their previous source was unreasonable; 73 percent of the medical patients expressed the same opinion.

Physician Accessibility and Emergency-Room Utilization

An important objective of GHS planners was to educate patients, particularly former clinic patients, to view GHS as a continuously available source of care, and thus to reduce their dependence on the hospital's emergency room. The interviewed patients were asked a series of questions relating to how they would go about getting help for themselves or for their children if a medical need suddenly became apparent at night or on Sunday. Their responses to what they would do under these circumstances are presented in table 6-9. The data show that, consistent with our earlier findings on actual emergency-room use, the pediatric sample of respondents were much more inclined to rely on GHS than were the medical sample. The parents of Genesee clinic patients were most likely to call GHS for help. By comparison, among medical respondents, the group of former clinic users were least likely to call GHS and most likely to go to an emergency room.

Several detailed questions concerning physician availability were asked.

Table 6-9
Course of Action in Emergency

	Previous Care Source		
Action Taken	Private	Clinic	Other
Pediatrics			
Call Genesee Health Service	69%	84%	59%
Phone doctor/exchange	13	5	8
Call police/ambulance	3	5	—
Call doctor and ambulance	—	—	3
Go to emergency room	15	—	28
Wait until morning/Monday	—	5	—
Don't know	—	—	3
	100%	100%	100%
Medicine			
Call Genesee Health Service	44%	32%	31%
Phone doctor/exchange	10	—	27
Call police/ambulance	10	16	—
Call doctor and ambulance	2	—	—
Go to emergency room	26	47	42
Wait until morning/Monday	—	—	—
Other	8	5	—
	100%	100%	100%

These data, which are presented in table 6-10, generally accord with opinions voiced in the community survey, but again we perceive a difference in attitude between the pediatric and the medical samples, with the former expressing greater confidence in the accessibility of their physician.

Table 6-10
Physician Accessibility

A Telephone Accessibility

"If you needed to reach a doctor on the phone at night or on Sunday, how much trouble do you think you would have—a great deal, some, or no trouble at all?"

	Pediatrics			Medicine		
Previous Source Of Care	Great Deal	Some Trouble	No Trouble	Great Deal	Some Trouble	No Trouble
Private	7%	19%	73%	18%	24%	56%
Genesee clinics	6	14	86	24	24	54
Other	15	24	62	30	16	55
Consumer survey	9	22	62	10	29	52

B House Calls

"Suppose you were so sick you needed a doctor to come to your house to examine you at night or on a Sunday. How much trouble do you think you would have getting a doctor to come to your house—a great deal, some, or no trouble at all?"

	Pediatrics			Medicine		
Previous Source Of Care	Great Deal	Some Trouble	No Trouble	Great Deal	Some Trouble	No Trouble
Private	49%	20%	31%	61%	17%	23%
Genesee clinics	28	36	36	41	27	33
Other	65	16	19	50	29	20
Consumer survey	52	24	24	51	25	24

C After-Hours Office Call

"Suppose you simply needed to see a doctor—but not to have him come to your home—and you were willing to go where he asked. How much trouble do you think you would have seeing a doctor at night or on Sunday—a great deal, some, or no trouble at all?"

	Pediatrics			Medicine		
Previous Source Of Care	Great Deal	Some Trouble	No Trouble	Great Deal	Some Trouble	No Trouble
Private	0%	24%	76%	17%	29%	54%
Genesee clinics	0	18	83	5	22	72
Other	10	27	64	27	31	42
Consumer survey	13	21	66	16	28	57

In the community survey, people provided widely divergent reasons for their utilization of a source of ambulatory care, depending on whether their medical need was urgent or not. For routine problems, quality of care factors predominated; for urgent problems, location of the emergency room was a principal factor in the choice. As the distance between alternative sources of care and residence increased, location became increasingly important. It is apparent from table 6-11 that the sample of GHS patients differed from the community sample in their perception of the importance of factors that caused them to select one emergency room over another. The patient's contact with GHS was relatively important, much more so than the general consumer's relationship with his regular source of care. This finding supports our suggestion in chapter 5 that, although a primary-care program may lessen the emergency-room use of its patients, the attraction of additional patients to the hospital is a countervailing factor that may lessen substantially the effect on total visits made to the hospital's own emergency facility.

The reductions in emergency-room utilization that we report in the previous chapter presumably are related primarily to use for nonurgent medical needs. For urgent medical problems, GHS patients chose a known, reliable, and accessible source when the urgency of the problem was a salient factor in their decision.

Table 6-11
Reasons for Patient Choice of Hospital Emergency Room
(*percent*)

| | Previous Source of Care | | | | | |
| | Pediatrics | | | Medicine | | |
Reason	Private	Clinic	Other	Private	Clinic	Other
Location	36	11	23	43	21	39
GHS affiliation[a]	36	32	46	23	37	19
Availability of competent physician	5	11	5	2	—	4
Previous experience	13	26	21	16	26	31
Efficiency of emergency room	8	16	3	14	11	4
Other[b]	2	4	2	2	5	3

[a]Associated with GHS, or doctor affiliated there, or next to GHS, or doctor said to go there.

[b]Family member or respondent employed there, know people there, transportation availability, insurance applicability, and appearance.

Acceptance of Physician Assistants

The maldistribution of ambulatory-care resources has prompted the greater use of paraprofessional personnel, such as physician assistants and nurse practitioners. To evaluate patient reaction to the use of such assistants, respondents were asked a series of questions similar to those asked in the community survey. To ensure that patients understood the meaning of the term, the questions were introduced with the following statement:

> Some doctors now use what are known as physician assistants — medical personnel with special training and expertise. They are qualified to treat many of the routine problems that people have. They also relieve the doctor of many of the tasks that don't require the greater expertise of the doctor; for example, performing routine aspects of physical examinations. They help to ensure that the doctor can see more quickly those patients who do need his attention.

Judging from table 6-12, both groups of GHS patients appeared willing to see a physician assistant in the office setting. However, parents in the pediatric sample were markedly less inclined to use the physician assistant

Table 6-12
Perceptions of the Use of Physician Assistants

A Willingness

"We'd like to know how willing you would be to see a physician assistant instead of a doctor in such circumstances. Would you be very willing, would you have doubts, or wouldn't you be willing at all?"

Sample	Very Willing	Have Doubts	Not Willing	Don't Know
GHS pediatrics	56%	26%	18%	—
GHS medicine	56	22	21	1%
Consumer survey	59	26	11	4

B Probability of Consultation

"If such a person were to become available for telephone conversation after normal working hours, is there considerable, some, a little, or no chance that you would call him rather than a doctor, should the need arise?"

Sample	Considerable	Some	A Little	No Chance	Don't Know
GHS pediatrics	33%	28%	12%	24%	3%
GHS medicine	50	24	9	17	1
Consumer survey	50	20	13	14	4

for telephone consultations than were either the medical patients or the respondents in the community survey. It is interesting to note that the parents had greater contact with the pediatric nurse practitioner than did medical patients with the physician assistant (31 versus 19 percent), so that their attitudes were not a consequence of less information or experience. But, when we examined patient attitudes while controlling for whether the respondent previously had experienced a contact with a physician assistant, we found that patients in both groups who had such an experience were much more inclined to either see or consult with one on the phone, than were patients who had no previous experience. Among medical patients, the willingness to deal with a physician assistant was much more apparent among males than females. In both samples, blacks were more willing than whites, notwithstanding that white patients had the greater contact with physician assistants, the more so in medicine than in pediatrics.

General Observations

Other questions in the survey yielded a variety of information, which we present without amplifying discussion:

1. The parents of pediatric patients were more aware of their doctor's name than were medical patients. Only 5 percent of the pediatric sample did not know the name of their child's doctor. For medicine, the figure was 14 percent.
2. Of the parents who used GHS for their child, 54 percent also used it for themselves.
3. Of the pediatric parents, 89 percent thought of their children's health "quite often," 9 percent "once in a while," 3 percent "hardly ever." For medicine the figures were 64, 22, and 14 percent, respectively.
4. Of the parents 53 percent discussed their children's health with family or friends "quite often"; 29 percent of the medical sample discussed their own health similarly.
5. Of the parents 80 percent took their children to a doctor regularly for check-ups, generally at least once a year. Of the medical patients 62 percent had regular check-ups. In comparison, 65 percent of the respondents in the consumer survey reported seeing a doctor regularly.

In our view, patient satisfaction is an important measure of the success of any endeavor to create a viable system of ambulatory health care. To this end, a variety of survey instruments were devised, all of which focused on eliciting from the consumer of health services his views on the standards of care delivery that were important to him. The consumer survey revealed that, in most instances, public perceptions of ambulatory care were in general agreement with the views of those who created the Genesee Health Service. Our study of GHS patients indicates that the new facility attracted a diverse patient population who, also, had similar views about health-care delivery. In the main, these people believe that GHS is a worthwhile alternative to other sources of care.

7 Goals, Findings, Qualifications, and Implications

Each year Americans make over one billion ambulatory-care visits. Of this total, one-fifth are made to hospital emergency rooms and clinics, for the most part by people who have no other readily available source of care. As sources of primary care, traditional hospital outpatient departments leave much to be desired. The episodic nature of patient visits and the usual absence of any continuously available primary-care physician makes it almost impossible to effect an ongoing management of patient problems. Paradoxically, it is the people who rely most on hospital facilities who need the most help in developing a planned approach to health care.

Goals

Genesee's planners were fully aware of the inadequacies of their hospital's ambulatory facilities. They felt obligated to provide a better system of care for their outpatient population. They also realized that any successful alternative to the clinics could have wide application in other hospitals. Their concept of a "better" system of care involved, primarily, a team of competent, accessible, and sympathetic providers, who would effect coordinated management of patient medical needs in a setting conductive to the creation of a warm doctor-patient relationship. They gave little emphasis to improving quality of care per se. Much more important in their view was an atmosphere that fostered the treatment of each patient with respect and dignity. As important to the ultimate success of the new system was its appeal to a large number of middle-class patients, who could bring needed financial stability to the program. This goal of a mixed patient population also was symbolic of the equity of opportunity that planners viewed as the philosophical foundation for their new health service. It was with these goals in mind that we formulated our research design. We required indicators of patterns of utilization, and we required a set of criteria with which to measure patient satisfaction with the health service. We also desired to create an evaluative model that could be used by other institutional planners.

121

We realized that health behavior is a complex phenomenon, but as we studied the literature we came to the conclusion that more often than not researchers had investigated the subject *in vacuo*. Virtually all human behavior is goal-oriented. Health-care behavior is causally related to the motivations that people have with respect to matters of health. But it is evident also that people have many non-health-related goals, and that these goals often conflict with decisions about their health. As a consequence, almost every health-related decision involves a tradeoff between competing wants and desires. This awareness prompted us to investigate the possible application of traditional theories of decision-making to the study of the Genesee Health Service.

We posited health behavior to be a process of rational choice, and we conceived of health-care utilization as a sequence of decisions that begin with the patient's perception of a medical problem or need. Subsequent decisions relate to the urgency of the problem or need, whether care should be sought, if so, what kind of care, and, finally, the choice of facility that under the circumstances seems to offer the greatest expected value. We argue that to understand patient utilization, we must know how the patient perceives the elements of these health-related decisions. We call these elements decision-components and, with respect to the choice of care facility, categorize them as economic, temporal, convenience, sociopsychological, and quality factors.

We conducted a community survey in order to identify the universe of things that matter to the patient's choice of care facility. With a simple algorithm, we calculated the respondent's rational choice of care and were able to document relatively high predictive efficacy of the respondent's reported volume source of care. In our view this established the validity and reliability of our use of these decision-components as evaluative criteria.

The second of our basic research tasks was to describe the hospital's outpatient population and, subsequently, the GHS population. We desired to describe the sociodemographic character of the population, and to document their utilization of hospital resources. With such data we intended to assess the extent to which GHS would be able to integrate those who traditionally have depended on hospitals for ambulatory care into a patient population more representative of the community as a whole. Heretofore researchers and hospital administrators have relied primarily on visit statistics for their planning needs. We viewed such data as essential, but limited and misleading in their usefulness, unless adjusted in some way to reflect the relationship with the patients by whom these visits are generated. We devised a method that permitted us to use these statistics to provide estimates of the hospital's outpatient population, and we eventually were able to create a profile of these patients and their utilization of hospital services, against which we later compared the GHS population.

Findings

Our studies provide several general findings. First, the data show that the Genesee Health Service has been accepted by the patient population for whom it was designed. The number of low-income, inner-city residents who receive primary-care services at the hospital has increased dramatically. Moreover, the health service also appeals to a large middle-income population, whose patronage was deemed necessary for its overall success.

Second, GHS was designed to be more accessible to its patient population than were the former outpatient clinics. The study of telephone utilization and the survey of GHS patients indicate that this goal has been achieved.

Third, the telephone data, the study of impact on the emergency room, and the study of preventive procedures in pediatrics demonstrate desirable changes in patient utilization behavior consistent with the health service's accessibility.

Fourth, patients who responded to our survey express greater satisfaction with GHS than with their former sources of care. This is true particularly of former clinic patients.

The generally positive findings of our studies must be tempered by several factors. While GHS has reduced the frequency of emergency-room visits by certain groups of its patients, because of the constraints of general utilization patterns it has not been able to effect a reduction in total emergency-room utilization that is significant administratively. Further, the impact of the program on patient behavior appears uneven across its specialties of pediatrics, medicine, and ob/gyn. Finally, although GHS does not seem to represent a particularly costly mode of care, the long-range financial prospects of it and similar programs remain unclear.[1]

Qualifications

While we certainly do not believe that the setting of the Genesee Health Service was unique in its basic character, several circumstances that furthered GHS development appear worthy of emphasis, lest we generalize too quickly from the experience. Although affiliated with the University of Rochester, Genesee is not a major teaching hospital. The freedom of planners to invoke changes in the delivery of care was no doubt greater than would have been possible at an institution where the interests of training programs, and the medical faculty responsible, predominate. We note that Genesee's residency program in ob/gyn was much stronger than in pediatrics or medicine, and the differences in the development and organization of the practices were readily apparent.[2]

The relative lack of emphasis on medical education at Genesee perhaps was a factor in the relatively small size of the outpatient specialty clinics. Moreover, as demonstrated by our profile of the emergency-room patient population, Genesee was not characteristic of a typical inner-city hospital on which a great number of patients depended as a regular source of ambulatory care. Whatever the reason, the clinics were of a manageable size that facilitated a smooth transition to the group practice.

The location of the hospital in a broadly accessible, reasonably pleasant area of the city appears to have aided in the attraction by GHS of additional middle-class patients. The availability of unused space in a modern professional building no doubt was a favorable circumstance, also. Finally, the acquisition of grant funds sufficient to construct a comfortable and attractive facility enabled GHS to advance its image as a locus of "private" practice.

Apart from the circumstantial qualifications pertinent to the development of GHS, our studies were limited in their objectives. We did not possess sufficient resources to examine longitudinally in detail the utilization patterns of the patient populations. And, for the most part, our descriptions of the populations are restricted to relatively short periods of time. Nor was it possible to examine closely the utilization that Genesee patients may have made of other local health facilities. It is reasonable to assume that multiple use of such facilities, particularly emergency rooms, did occur. Further, the impact of GHS on the Rochester community, as viewed by that community, remains outside our purview.[3]

Implications

Whatever were the circumstances that benefited the Genesee Health Service, probably just as many favored the status quo. Thus, the program could not have been successful without the firm commitment of Genesee's administration and many of its medical staff to create a more desirable alternative to the existing clinics. Of equal importance was the management skill necessary to carry through this major endeavor. Judging from the patient survey, GHS developers were effective in creating a service that appeals to a broad segment of the community. The aesthetic appearance of the facility, the attitude of the staff, the concept of continuity of care, and the geographic and temporal accessibility of the health service all helped to attract a broad mix of patients. Perhaps as important was the manner in which physician staff were recruited. The early acquisition of several local physicians with established practices provided an initial influx of middle-class patients. The presence of these patients and the physical characteristics of the facility helped to create the image of a private practice with which prospective patients readily could associate. As additional physicians joined GHS, the phased referrrals of clinic patients helped them develop their practices at a comfortable pace. Thus, not only was the goal of a mixed patient population achieved, but the manner in which this was accomplished provided momentum for the subsequent rapid growth in patient volume.

To those involved in the planning of health-care delivery, the most encouraging aspect of our findings is the performance of the GHS pediatric group, whose willingness to assume responsibility for the continuous management of care appears to have been accepted by parents on a broad basis. In explaining the somewhat lesser impact of GHS on adult health behavior, we suggest that the maturity and experience of the person who makes the decision to seek care may be particularly important. An adult usually decides for himself about matters relating to health care, but parents decide for their children. Since the parent cannot know how a child actually feels, there is greater uncertainty about the seriousness of a problem and the proper course of action. Given access to a primary-care physician, a parent may be more readily inclined to contact the physician and obtain advice, before going to an emergency room. Conversely, an adult may be certain of the need for immediate medical attention and, therefore, may be less inclined to take the trouble first to contact the physician.

In our view the success of any effort to create an acceptable and viable ambulatory-care program can be measured usefully in terms of patient satisfaction. Our analysis of data from the survey of GHS patients and the documented growth of the new service suggest that it has been a success. Yet, these findings must be qualified because of the difficulty that we encountered in locating inner-city patients for interviews. An earlier effort to locate and interview former outpatient-clinic patients was singularly unsuccessful. In that exercise, we dismissed the problem as a consequence of poor recordkeeping and old patient data. Following the survey experience, we must reevaluate that conclusion. In two of our studies, notwithstanding considerable investigative efforts, prospective inner-city respondents simply could not be located.

Given the problems that we experienced in locating a specified group of patients, it would seem unwise to design an inner-city health-care facility to serve only a stable target population. The transient characteristics of inner-city people are likely to generate a demand for episodic care, and much greater need, albeit unsolicited, for preventive care. Medical record data for these patients will be incomplete. Compliance probably will be poor. Moreover, all of these problems will be common to each institution or facility. Clearly these matters reinforce the need for coordinated community planning and for some form of comprehensive, computerized medical information system that would be accessible to any facility to which the patient may turn for care. Given proper assurance of confidentiality, each facility could, as appropriate, add to the patient's record, thereby making available up-to-date information to any subsequent provider.

In addition to enhancing continuity of care, a comprehensive medical information system would enable our study of utilization at Genesee to be replicated on a larger scale. Such data are necessary in order to understand fully the use of community resources by a population, in particular the use of multiple resources by the same persons. Each institution's planners tend to think of their own institution independently of others. However, without knowledge of how people use different facilities, planning an efficient strategy to meet overall community needs is almost impossible. Until we understand more about what motivates individual health behavior, we cannot reliably predict future requirements.[4]

If one cannot change the nature of consumer demand or of health-related behavior, then it might be wise to redesign the system of delivery to serve existing demand more efficiently. This is not to say that efforts such as GHS are in vain. GHS planners have demonstrated that within the inner-city community are many people who desire more than episodic care. But it is also false to assume that all former clinic patients view the new health service as a more desirable alternative to the hospital's old outpatient facility. About one-third of the small group of patients in the GHS survey who reported leaving the health service indicated that they were using instead a neighborhood health center, another hospital's clinics, or an emergency room for the treatment of their medical problems. Apparently, the wants and desires of these people were not fulfilled at GHS.

The satisfaction of some patients with what others would argue are less desirable alternatives clearly reflects their possession of a different set of values, which in our view makes their choice of these other facilities *rational*, as we define the term. But how do we account for these differences among people? The likely explanation is that people are a product of their environment. Patients who over the years have been socialized to accept the impersonal care of the hospital clinic may feel uncomfortable in the very different surroundings of the private office setting. Similarly, although deemed desirable by health-care planners, some people do not want to see the same doctor every time they need health-care treatment or advice. Some people place great value on anonymity and view the questions of well-meaning staff as an instrusion on their privacy. Some patients do not desire even an efficient appointment system. In our interviews with clinic users, we found some elderly patients for whom time had little value and for whom the medical visit represented an encounter with other people that was altogether too infrequent. To them the visit was a social occasion, to be savored with anticipation as a rare break in the otherwise dull monotony of their lives. They did not desire an appointment system, because they had no interest in decreasing their time spent waiting to see the physician. But, allowing for such exceptions, in the main we found that people appreciate Genesee's new program of ambulatory care.

It is argued that, as a consequence of a lifelong intimate association with the most deleterious aspects of our society, the poor have the most deeply ingrained and most undesirable health habits. It would seem that these habits are merely a learned response to their environment. Our evaluation of the Genesee Health Service has demonstrated that when people are provided with an alternative source of care, many accept and comply with a pattern of utilization deemed more desirable by health professionals. Genesee's planners have shown that a better system of urban health-care delivery can be designed, and that community hospitals can play a major role in improving the well-being of inner-city people.

Notes

1. The financial and organizational implications of hospital-sponsored group practice may become clearer as a result of a study being conducted on a large group of programs developed subsequently to the Genesee Health Service. See Stephen M. Shortell et al., "Hospital Sponsored Primary Care: Organizational and Financial Issues," *Medical Group Management* vol. 25, no. 3 (May-June 1978):16.

2. The GHS ob/gyn component is described in detail by Robert C. Tatelbaum and Donna I. Regenstreif, "An Ambulatory Training Model for an Obstetrics and Gynecology Residency Program," *Journal of Medical Education* 53(1978):344. The development of group practices in teaching hospitals is discussed by Arthur A. Berarducci, Thomas L. Delbanco, and Mitchell T. Rabkin, "The Teaching Hospital and Primary Care: Closing Down the Clinics," *New England Journal of Medicine* 292(1975):615; and Jerome H. Grossman, John D. Stoeckle, and James J. Dineen, "New Organizations Out of Old Ones: Teaching Group Practices Out of Private Practices and Outpatient Departments," *Milbank Memorial Fund Quarterly* 53(1975):65. A candid portrayal of group practice development at a medical school is presented by Gerald T. Perkoff, *Changing Health Care: Perspectives from a New Medical Setting* (Ann Arbor, Mich.: Health Administration Press, 1979).

3. A research design for evaluating the impact that hospital-sponsored group practices have on access to medical care in their communities is described by Ronald Andersen et al., "Overview of a Design to Evaluate the Impact of Community Hospital-Sponsored Primary Care Group Practices," *Medical Group Management* vol. 25, no. 5 (September-October 1978):16.

4. See the discussion concerning emergency-room services in William C. Stratmann and Ralph Ullman, "A Study of Consumer Attitudes about Health Care: The Role of the Emergency Room," *Medical Care* 13(1975):1033.

Appendix:
Community Survey
Questionnaire

Good _____ .   I'm _____ of _____.

We are trying to get a clearer picture of the health care needs in the

greater Rochester area.   In this interview, we are particularly interested

in your views on the health care which you are now receiving.   We will

be asking you about where you go for health care services, why you go to

that particular place, and how you feel about the way you are treated there.

Your answers will be held in strict confidence and no one will be

able to tell which answers are yours and which were given by others.

Please answer only for yourself and not for other members of your family,

except where the question asks about other members of your family.

Time Interview Began _____

la. Is there any one place or person that you feel you can rely upon

when you need help about a medical problem?   Is there someone or

some one place that you feel you can always turn to when you need

medical help or advice?

Yes   1

No   5   (SKIP TO #2a)

b. (HAND RESPONDENT CARD "A") Would it involve going to one of these

five places?

Yes   1   (ASK #1c AND SKIP TO #1e)

No   5   (SKIP TO #1d)

_____

Note to reader: The Rochester Survey was conducted by a professional research firm. The
questionnaire used makes reference to a Master Sheet on which interviews summarized respondent reasons for using one facility or another (what we define as decision-components). The
Master Sheet was also used to document the relative importance of these factors to the respondent, and, for alternative sources, the satisfaction he might expect to receive with respect to
each factor. A copy of the Master Sheet is provided at the end of the questionnaire.

c. Which one?

                    Hospital Emergency Room 1

                    Hospital Clinic 2

                    Private Doctor's Office 3

                    Clinic at Work 4

                    Neighborhood Health Center 5

d. What type of place would it involve going to? _____

e. If for any reason this place were not available to you, to which

    of these (other) places would you go instead?

                    Hospital Emergency Room 1

                    Hospital Clinic 2

                    Private Doctor's Office 3

                    Clinic at Work 4

                    Neighborhood Health Center 5

                    None of These 6

                    Don't Know 8

2a. (HAND RESPONDENT CARD "A" IF "NO" TO #1a) Now I'm going to ask you

     some questions about each of these types of places; first of all,

     the Hospital Emergency Room. Some people have been to a Hospital

     Emergency Room as a result of a serious accident in which they were

     injured and needed immediate medical assistance. Other people

     use Hospital Emergency Rooms by choice for help with either urgent

     medical problems or ordinary-routine medical problems or both.

     Have you ever been to a Hospital Emergency Room of your own choice

     for either an urgent or an ordinary-routine problem?

                    Yes   1   (CHECK "YES" ON MASTER SHEET FOR HOSP.EMER. &

                                SKIP TO 2c)

                    No   5   (ASK #2b AND SKIP TO #5a)

b. Why haven't you ever gone to a Hospital Emergency Room of your own
    choice?

    (MAKE NOTES HERE.   THEN RECORD REASONS ON MASTER SHEET)

c. Was it for an urgent problem, an ordinary-routine problem, or both?

                Urgent Problem   1

                Ordinary-Routine Problem   3

                Both   5

2d. Which Hospital Emergency Room in the Rochester Area do you usually
    go to? _____

    (IF UNABLE TO ANSWER) Which did you go to most recently? _____

e. Have you ever been to any others in the Rochester Area?

                Yes   1

                No   5   (SKIP TO #3a)

f. Which one or ones? _____

g. Which one(s) wouldn't you go to again? _____

h. Why wouldn't you go to (this/these) Hospital Emergency Room(s)
    again?

    (MAKE NOTES HERE.   THEN RECORD REASONS ON MASTER SHEET)

3a. How many years ago did you first go to the   (#2d)   Hospital
    Emergency Room? _____

b. How did you first hear about the services available at the   (#2d)
    Hospital Emergency Room?

    _____

    _____

    _____

c. What was it you heard that made you decide to go there, rather
    than somewhere else?
    (MAKE NOTES HERE.   THEN RECORD REASONS ON MASTER SHEET)

d. What do you like about the __(#2d)__ Hospital Emergency Room?

(MAKE NOTES HERE. THEN RECORD REASONS ON MASTER SHEET)

e. What do you dislike about the __(#2d)__ Hospital Emergency Room?

(MAKE NOTES HERE. THEN RECORD REASONS ON MASTER SHEET)

3f. When you go to a Hospital Emergency Room, is the problem usually

so urgent that you have to see a doctor right away, or can you

usually wait a while and put off seeing him until the next day?

Urgent 1

Can Wait a While 5

g. Have you ever had difficulty talking to the staff of a Hospital

Emergency Room because of language problems?

Yes   1

No   5

4a. Have you been to a Hospital Emergency Room in the Rochester Area

for medical help or advice within the past 12 months?

Yes   1

No   5

b. (HAND MALE RESPONDENTS BLUE CARD "B" AND FEMALE RESPONDENTS PINK

CARD "B") Here is a list of reasons for people seeking medical

help or advice. Which of these have been reasons for your going

to a Hospital Emergency Room during the past 12 months? (CHECK

UNDER "b" BELOW)

c. (FOR EACH REASON CHECKED "YES") How many times have you been to a

local Hospital Emergency Room during the past 12 months _____?

(RECORD UNDER "c" BELOW)

d. (FOR EACH REASON CHECKED "YES") What type or types of doctors did

you see _____? (RECORD UNDER "d" BELOW)

	"b" Reason? Yes No	"c" No. of Times	"d" Type(s) of Doctor
For a Checkup	1 5	_____	_____
For Other Ordinary-Routine Problems	1 5	_____	_____
For Inoculation	1 5	_____	_____
For an Urgent Problem Requiring Immediate Medical Attention .	1 5	_____	_____
Because of Pregnancy	1 5	_____	_____
Because of "Female Problems"...	1* 5	_____	_____
For All Other Reasons	1 5	_____	_____

* CHECK "YES" ON MASTER SHEET

5a. The second place listed on Card "A" is the Hospital Clinic. Have you
   ever gone to a Hospital Clinic in the Rochester Area for medical
   help or advice?

   Yes   1   (CHECK "YES" ON MASTER SHEET FOR HOS.CLIN.&

   SKIP TO 5c)

   No   5   (ASK #5b AND SKIP TO #8a)

b. Why haven't you ever gone to a Hospital Clinic for a medical problem?
   (MAKE NOTES HERE. THEN RECORD REASONS ON MASTER SHEET)

c. Which Hospital Clinic in the Rochester Area do you usually go to?

   _____

   (IF UNABLE TO ANSWER) Which did you go to most recently?

   _____

d. Have you ever been to any others in the Rochester Area?

Yes   1

No   5   (SKIP TO #6a)

e. Which one or ones? _____

f. Which one(s) wouldn't you go to again? _____

5g. Why wouldn't you go to (this/these) Hospital Clinic(s) again?

(MAKE NOTES HERE. THEN RECORD REASONS ON MASTER SHEET)

6a. How many years ago did you first go to the (#5c) Hospital Clinic?

b. How did you first hear about the services available at the (#5c)

Hospital Clinic?

_____

_____

_____

c. What was it you heard that made you decide to go there, rather than

some place else?

(MAKE NOTES HERE. THEN RECORD REASONS ON MASTER SHEET)

d. What do you like about the (#5c) Hospital Clinic?

(MAKE NOTES HERE. THEN RECORD REASONS ON MASTER SHEET)

e. What do you dislike about the (#5c) Hospital Clinic?

(MAKE NOTES HERE. THEN RECORD REASONS ON MASTER SHEET)

f. When you go to a Hospital Clinic, is the problem usually so urgent

that you have to see a doctor right away, or can you usually wait

a while and put of seeing him until the next day?

Urgent 1

Can Wait a While 5

g. Have you ever had difficulty talking to the staff of a Hospital

Clinic because of language problems?

        Yes   1

        No   5

7a. Have you been to a Hospital Clinic in the Rochester Area within the

past 12 months?

        Yes   1

        No   5   (SKIP TO #8a)

7b. (IF NOT PREVIOUSLY USED, HAND MALE RESPONDENTS BLUE CARD "B" AND

FEMALE RESPONDENTS PINK CARD "B" AND SAY: "Here is a list of

reasons for people seeking medical help or advice.") Which of the

reasons listed on Card "B" are reasons for your going to a Hospital

Clinic during the past 12 months?

(CHECK UNDER "b" BELOW)

c. (FOR EACH REASON CHECKED "YES") How many times have you been to a

local Hospital Clinic during the past 12 months _____?

(RECORD UNDER "c" BELOW)

d. (FOR EACH REASON CHECKED "YES") What type of doctor did you see

_____? (RECORD UNDER "d" BELOW)

	"b"		"c"	"d"
	Reason?		No. of	
	Yes	No	Times	Type(s) of Doctor
For a Checkup	1	5	_____	_____
For Other Ordinary-Routine Problems	1	5	_____	_____
For Inoculations	1	5	_____	_____
For an Urgent Problem Requiring Immediate Medical Attention .	1	5	_____	_____

Because of Pregnancy 1   5   _____ _____

Because of "Female Problems"... 1*   5   _____ _____

For All Other Reasons 1   5   _____ _____

* CHECK "YES" ON MASTER SHEET IF NOT ALREADY CHECKED.

8a. The third place listed on Card "A" is the Private Doctor's Office.

Have you ever visited a Private Doctor in the Rochester Area, at his

or her office, for medical help or advice?

> Yes   1   (CHECK "YES" ON MASTER SHEET FOR DOCTOR &
>
> SKIP TO 8c)
>
> No   5   (ASK #8b AND SKIP TO #18a)

b. Why have you never visited a Private Doctor?

(MAKE NOTES HERE. THEN RECORD REASONS ON MASTER SHEET)

c. (HAND MALE RESPONDENTS BLUE CARD "C" AND FEMALE RESPONDENTS PINK

CARD "C") Here is a list of types of doctors. Which of these have

have you ever visited at their private offices in the Rochester

Area for medical help or advice? (CHECK UNDER "c" BELOW)

d. (IF TWO OR MORE CHECKED "YES") Which of these types have you

visited most in their private offices? (RECORD "FIRST" UNDER "d"

BELOW)

(IF THREE OR MORE CHECKED "YES") Which would be next? (RECORD

"SECOND" UNDER "d" BELOW)

(IF FOUR OR MORE CHECKED "YES") Which would be next ? (RECORD

"THIRD" UNDER "d" BELOW)

NOTE: IF ONLY ONE IS CHECKED "YES", RECORD "FIRST" UNDER "d"

OPPOSITE IT. IF THREE ARE CHECKED "YES", RECORD "THIRD"

UNDER "d" FOR THE ONE NOT ALREADY RANKED.

	"c"		"d"
	Visited?		
	Yes	No	_____ Rank _____
General Practitioner	1	5	_____
Internist	1	5	_____
Ophthalmologist	1	5	_____
Gynecologist	1	5	_____
Obstetrician	1	5	_____
Medical Specialist	1	5	_____
Other	1	5	_____

(IF "FIRST" ONLY, ASK 9 - 11 AND SKIP TO #18a.)

(IF "FIRST" AND "SECOND" ONLY, ASK 9 - 14 AND SKIP TO #18a.)

9a. How many private __(First in #8d)__ s have you gone to in the

Rochester Area for medical help or advice? _____

(IF "1", SKIP TO #10a)

b. Are there any private __(First in #8d)__ s that you wouldn't go to

again?

                    Yes   1

                    No   5   (SKIP TO #10a)

c. Why wouldn't you go to (this/these) private __(First in #8d)__ (s)

again?

(MAKE NOTES HERE. THEN RECORD REASONS ON MASTER SHEET)

10a. How many years ago did you first go to the private __(First in #8d)__

you usually visit? _____ years.

(IF UNABLE TO ANSWER) How many years ago did you first go to the

private __(First in #8d)__ you visited most recently? _____ years.

b. How did you first hear about this doctor? _____

_____

_____

_____

c. What was it you heard that made you decide to see him, rather than
    someone else?

    (MAKE NOTES HERE. THEN RECORD ON MASTER SHEET)

d. What do you like about this ___(First in #8d)___, or about his or her
    office, equipment, facilities, staff, etc. ?

    (MAKE NOTES HERE. THEN RECORD REASONS ON MASTER SHEET)

e. What do you dislike about this doctor, or about his or her office,
    equipment, facilities, staff, etc.?

    (MAKE NOTES HERE. THEN RECORD REASONS ON MASTER SHEET)

f. When you go to this doctor, is the problem usually so urgent that
    you have to see the doctor right away, or can you usually wait a
    while and put off seeing him until the next day?

                    Urgent 1

                    Can Wait a While 5

11a. Have you been to a private ___(First in #8d)___ in the Rochester Area
     within the past 12 months?

                    Yes   1

                    No   5   (SKIP TO #12a OR #18a, WHICHEVER APPLIES)

b. (IF NOT PREVIOUSLY USED, HAND MALE RESPONDENTS BLUE CARD "B" AND
    FEMALE RESPONDENTS PINK CARD "B" AND SAY: "Here is a list of
    reasons for people seeking medical help or advice.") Which of the
    reasons listed on Card "B" are reasons for your going to a local
    private ___(First in #8d)___ during the past 12 months?

    (CHECK UNDER "b" BELOW)

c.   (FOR EACH REASON CHECKED "YES") How many times have you been to a

local private ___(First in #8d)___ during the past 12 months _____?

(RECORD UNDER "c" BELOW)

	"b" Reason?		"c" No. of
	Yes	No	Times
For a Checkup	1	5	_____
For Other Ordinary-Routine Problems	1	5	_____
For an Urgent Problem Requiring Immediate Medical Attention.	1	5	_____
Because of Pregnancy	1	5	_____
Because of "Female Problems" ..	1*	5	_____
For All Other Reasons	1	5	_____

* CHECK "YES" ON MASTER SHEET IF NOT ALREADY CHECKED.

12a. How many private ___(Second in #8d)___ s have you gone to in the

Rochester Area for medical help or advice?

_____ (IF "1", SKIP TO #13a)

b.   Are there any private ___(Second in #8d)___ s that you wouldn't go to

again?

        Yes   1

        No   5   (SKIP TO #13a)

c.   Why wouldn't you go to (this/these) private ___(Second in #8d)___

again?

(MAKE NOTES HERE. THEN RECORD REASONS ON MASTER SHEET)

13a. How many years ago did you first go to the private (Second in #8d)

you usually visit?   _____ years

(IF UNABLE TO ANSWER) How many years ago did you first go to the private ___(Second in #8d)___ you visited most recently?

_____ years.

b. How did you first hear about this doctor? _____

_____

_____

_____

c. What was it you heard that made you decide to see him, rather than to see someone else?

(MAKE NOTES HERE. THEN RECORD REASONS ON MASTER SHEET)

13d. What do you like about this ___(Second in #8d)___ , or about his or her office, equipment, facilities, staff, etc.?

(MAKE NOTES HERE. THEN RECORD REASONS ON MASTER SHEET)

e. What do you dislike about this doctor, or about his or her office, equipment, facilities, staff, etc.?

(MAKE NOTES HERE. THEN RECORD REASONS ON MASTER SHEET)

f. When you go to this doctor, is the problem usually so urgent that you have to see the doctor right away, or can you usually wait a while and put off seeing him until the next day?

Urgent 1

Can Wait a While 5

14a. Have you been to a private ___(Second in #8d)___ in the Rochester Area within the past 12 months?

Yes   1

No   5   (SKIP TO #15a OR #18a, WHICHEVER APPLIES)

b. (REFER TO CARD "B") Which of the reasons listed on Card "B" are
    reasons for your going to a local private (Second in #8d)
    during the past 12 months? (CHECK UNDER "b" BELOW)

c. (FOR EACH REASON CHECKED "YES") How many times have you been to a
    local private (Second in #8d)   during the past 12 months_____?
    (RECORD UNDER "c" BELOW)

	"b"		"c"
	Reason?		No. of
	Yes	No	Times
For a Checkup	1	5	_____
For Other Ordinary-Routine			
Problems	1	5	_____
For Inoculations	1	5	_____
For an Urgent Problem Requiring			
Immediate Medical Attention.	1	5	_____
Because of Pregnancy	1	5	_____
Because of "Female Problems"...	1*	5	_____
For All Other Reasons	1	5	_____

* CHECK "YES" ON MASTER SHEET IF NOT ALREADY CHECKED.

15a. How many private (Third in #8d)   s have you gone to in the Rochester
     Area for medical help or advice? _____ (IF "1", SKIP TO #16a)

b. Are there any private (Third in #8d)   s that you wouldn't go to
    again?

                    Yes   1

                    No   5 (SKIP TO #16a)

c. Why wouldn't you go to (this/these) private (Third in #8d)   s
    again?

    (MAKE NOTES HERE. THEN RECORD REASONS ON MASTER SHEET)

16a. How many years ago did you first go to the private (Third in #8d)

you usually visit? _____ years

(IF UNABLE TO ANSWER) How many years ago did you first go to the

private (Third in #8d)   you visited most recently?

_____ years

b. How did you first hear about this doctor? _____

_____   _____

_____

_____

c. What was it you heard that made you decide to see him, rather than

to see someone else?

(MAKE NOTES HERE. THEN RECORD REASONS ON MASTER SHEET)

d. What do you like about this doctor, or about his or her office,

equipment, facilities, staff, etc.?

(MAKE NOTES HERE. THEN RECORD REASONS ON MASTER SHEET)

e. What do you dislike about this doctor, or about his or her office,

equipment, facilities, staff, etc.?

(MAKE NOTES HERE. THEN RECORD REASONS ON MASTER SHEET)

f. When you go to this doctor, is the problem usually so urgent that

you have to see the doctor right away, or can you usually wait a

while and put off seeing him until the next day?

Urgent 1

Can Wait a While 5

17a. Have you been to a private (Third in #8d)   in the Rochester Area

within the past 12 months?

Yes   1

No   5 (SKIP TO #18a)

17b. (REFER TO CARD "B") Which of the reasons listed on Card "B" are

reasons for your going to a private (Third in #8d) during the

past 12 months? (CHECK UNDER "b" BELOW)

c. (FOR EACH REASON CHECKED "YES") How many times have you been to a

local private (Third in #8d) during the past 12 months _____?

(RECORD UNDER "c" BELOW)

	"b"		"c"
	Reason?		No. of
	Yes	No	Times
For a Checkup	1	5	_____
For Other Ordinary-Routine			
Problems	1	5	_____
For Inoculations	1	5	_____
For an Urgent Problem Requiring			
Immediate Medical Attention.	1	5	_____
Because of Pregnancy	1	5	_____
Because of "Female Problems" ..	1 *	5	_____
For All Other Reasons	1	5	_____

* CHECK "YES" ON MASTER SHEET IF NOT ALREADY CHECKED.

18a. The fourth place listed on Card "A" is the Clinic at Work. Have

you ever worked for a company in the Rochester Area that maintains

a medical clinic?

        Yes   1

        No   5 (SKIP TO #21a)

b. Have you ever voluntarily used such a clinic?

        Yes   1 (CHECK "YES" ON MASTER SHEET FOR CLINIC

                       AT WORK & SKIP TO #19a.)

        No   5 (ASK #18c AND SKIP TO #21a)

c. Why not?

(MAKE NOTES HERE. THEN RECORD REASONS ON MASTER SHEET)

19a. Which company's medical clinic did you go to most recently?

_____

  b. What was it you heard about the clinic that made you decide to
go there, rather than to some place else?

(MAKE NOTES HERE. THEN RECORD REASONS ON MASTER SHEET)

  c. What do you like about the _____ clinic?

(MAKE NOTES HERE. THEN RECORD REASONS ON MASTER SHEET)

  d. What do you dislike about the _____ clinic?

(MAKE NOTES HERE. THEN RECORD REASONS ON MASTER SHEET)

19e. When you go to a Clinic at Work, is the problem usually so urgent
that you have to see a doctor right away, or can you usually wait
a while and put off seeing him until the next day?

Urgent..................... 1

Can Wait 5

20a. Have you been to a Clinic at Work in the Rochester Area within the
past 12 months?

Yes   1

No   5   (SKIP TO #21a)

  b. (IF NOT PREVIOUSLY USED, HAND MALE RESPONDENTS BLUE CARD "B" AND
FEMALE RESPONDENTS PINK CARD "B" AND SAY: "Here is a list of
reasons for people seeking medical help or advice.") Which of the
reasons listed on Card "B" are reasons for your going to a Clinic
at Work during the past 12 months? (CHECK UNDER "b" BELOW)

c.   (FOR EACH REASON CHECKED "YES") How many times have you been to

a Clinic at Work during the past 12 months _____?

(RECORD UNDER "c" BELOW)

	"b" Reason?		"c" No. of
	Yes	No	Times
For a Checkup	1	5	_____
For Other Ordinary-Routine Problems	1	5	_____
For Inoculations	1	5	_____
For an Urgent Problem Requiring Immediate Medical Attention.	1	5	_____
Because of Pregnancy	1	5	_____
Because of "Female Problems" ..	1*	5	_____
For All Other Reasons	1	5	_____

* CHECK "YES" ON MASTER SHEET IF NOT ALREADY CHECKED.

21a.   The fifth and last place listed on Card "A" is the Neighborhood

Health Center. Have you ever gone to a Neighborhood Health

Center in the Rochester Area for medical help or advice?

Yes   1   (CHECK "YES" ON MASTER SHEET FOR HEALTH CN. &

SKIP TO #21c.)

No   5   (ASK #21b AND SKIP TO #24a)

b.   Why have you never gone to a Neighborhood Health Center?

(MAKE NOTES HERE. THEN RECORD REASONS ON MASTER SHEET)

c.   Which Neighborhood Health Center in the Rochester Area do you

usually go to?   _____

(IF UNABLE TO ANSWER) Which did you go to most recently?

_____

d.   Have you ever been to any others in the Rochester Area?

        Yes   1

        No   5   (SKIP TO #22a)

e.   Which one or ones?   _____

f.   Which one(s) wouldn't you go to again?   _____

21g.   Why wouldn't you go to (this/these) Neighborhood Health Center(s) again?

     (MAKE NOTES HERE.   THEN RECORD REASONS ON MASTER SHEET)

22a.   How many years ago did you first go to the   (#21c)   Neighborhood Health Center?   _____ years.

b.   How did you first hear about the services available at the (#21c) Neighborhood Health Center? _____

_____

_____

c.   What was it you heard that made you decide to go there, rather than to some place else?

     (MAKE NOTES HERE.   THEN RECORD REASONS ON MASTER SHEET)

d.   What do you like about the   (#21c)   Neighborhood Health Center?

     (MAKE NOTES HERE.   THEN RECORD REASONS ON MASTER SHEET)

e.   What do you dislike about the   (#21c)   Neighborhood Health Center?

     (MAKE NOTES HERE.   THEN RECORD REASONS ON MASTER SHEET)

f.   When you go to a Neighborhood Health Center, is the problem usually so urgent that you have to see a doctor right away, or can you usually wait a while and put off seeing him until the next day?

                          Urgent 1

                          Can Wait a While 5

g.   Have you ever had difficulty talking to the staff of a Neighborhood

      Health Center because of language problems?

                    Yes   1

                    No   5

23a. Have you been to a Neighborhood Health Center in the Rochester

      Area within the past 12 months?

                    Yes   1

                    No   5   (SKIP TO #24a)

23b. (IF NOT PREVIOUSLY USED, HAND MALE RESPONDENTS BLUE CARD "B"

      AND FEMALE RESPONDENTS PINK CARD "B" AND SAY: "Here is a list

      of reasons for people seeking medical help or advice.")   Which

      of the reasons listed on Card "B" are reasons for your going to

      a Neighborhood Health Center during the past 12 months?

      (CHECK UNDER "b" BELOW)

c.   (FOR EACH REASON CHECKED "YES") How many times have you been to

      a local Neighborhood Health Center during the past 12 months_____?

      (RECORD UNDER "c" BELOW)

d.   (FOR EACH REASON CHECKED "YES") What type or types of doctor did

      you see _____? (RECORD UNDER "d" BELOW)

		"b"		"c"	"d"
		Reason?		No. of	
		Yes	No	Times	Type(s) of Doctor
For a Checkup		1	5	_____	_____
For Other Ordinary-Routine					
Problems		1	5	_____	_____
For Inoculations		1	5	_____	_____

For an Urgent Problem Requiring

    Immediate Medical Attention. 1   5   _____ _____

Because of Pregnancy 1   5   _____ _____

Because of "Female Problems"... 1*   5   _____ _____

For All Other Reasons 1   5   _____ _____

* CHECK "YES" ON MASTER SHEET IF NOT ALREADY CHECKED.

24a. Are there any children under 18 living in this household at the
present time?

        Yes   1

        No   5   (SKIP TO #29a AND THEN TO #34a)

b. How many are there? _____

c. How many are boys and how many are girls? Boys ____ Girls ____

d. Do you usually take (him/her/any of them) for medical care or
does someone else in the household usually do that?

        Respondent 1   (CHECK "YES" ON MASTER SHEET

                          FOR CHILDREN)

        Someone else 5   (SKIP TO #29a)

25a. (REFER TO CARD "A") To which of the places in the Rochester Area
listed on Card "A" do you usually take (him/her/them) for ordinary-
routine problems?

        Hospital Emergency Room 1

        Hospital Clinic 2

        Private Doctor's Office 3

        Clinic at Work 4

        Neighborhood Health Center 5

        (EACH PLACE CHECKED MUST ALSO BE CHECKED

        "YES" ON MASTER SHEET)

b. Is there any other place listed on this card in the Rochester
Area to which you used to take (him/her/them) but no longer do?

Yes   1

No   5   (SKIP TO #26a)

c.   Which place is this?

                   Hospital Emergency Room 1

                   Hospital Clinic 2

                   Private Doctor's Office 3

                   Clinic at Work 4

                   Neighborhood Health Center 5

              (EACH PLACE CHECKED MUST ALSO BE CHECKED

              "YES" ON MASTER SHEET)

d.   Why do you no longer take (him/her/them) to a ___(#25c)___ ?
     (MAKE NOTES HERE. THEN RECORD REASONS ON MASTER SHEET)

26a. (IF "PRIVATE DOCTOR'S OFFICE" TO #25a, SKIP TO #26b) Getting

      back to where you usually take (him/her/them), which (hospital/

      company/health center) is that? _____

b.   What type of doctor do you usually take (him/her/them) to?

     _____

c.   Is there another ___(#25a)___ in the Rochester Area to which you

     used to take (him/her/them) but no longer do?

                   Yes   1

                   No   5   (SKIP TO #27a)

d.   Why do you no longer take (him/her/them) to this ___(#25a)___ ?
     (MAKE NOTES HERE. THEN RECORD REASONS ON MASTER SHEET)

27a. How many years ago did you first take (him/her/them) to the

      ___(#25a)___ you do?   _____ _____ years.

b.   How did you first hear about this ___(#25a)___ ? _____

     _____

     _____

c.   What was it you heard that made you decide to go there, rather than to some place else?

(MAKE NOTES HERE. THEN RECORD REASONS ON MASTER SHEET)

d.   What do you like about this ___(#25a)___ ?

(MAKE NOTES HERE. THEN RECORD REASONS ON MASTER SHEET)

e.   What do you dislike about this ___(#25a)___ ?

(MAKE NOTES HERE. THEN RECORD REASONS ON MASTER SHEET)

27f.   When you take (him/her/them) is the problem usually so urgent that you have to see a doctor right away, or can you usually wait a while and put off seeing him until the next day?

           Urgent 1

           Can Wait a While 5

28a.   Have you taken (him/her/them) for medical care within the past 12 months in the Rochester Area?

           Yes   1

           No   5   (SKIP TO #29a)

b.   (REFER FEMALE RESPONDENTS TO PINK CARD "B" AND HAND MALE RESPON-DENTS PINK CARD "B" IF A GIRL IS INVOLVED) Which of these have been reasons for your taking (him/her/them) for medical care during the past 12 months? (CHECK UNDER "b" BELOW)

c.   (FOR EACH REASON CHECKED "YES") How many times have you taken (him/her/them) during the past 12 months _____?

(RECORD UNDER "c" BELOW)

d.   (FOR EACH REASON CHECKED "YES") What type or types of doctors did you see _____? (RECORD UNDER "d" BELOW)

	"b"		"c"	"d"
	Reason?		No. of	
	'Yes	No	Times	Type(s) of Doctor
For a Checkup	1	5	_____	_____
For Other Ordinary-Routine				
Problems	1	5	_____	_____
For Inoculations	1	5	_____	_____
For an Urgent Problem Requiring				
Immediate Medical Attention.	1	5	_____	_____
Because of Pregnancy	1	5	_____	_____
Because of "Female Problems" ..	1	5	_____	_____
For All Other Reasons	1	5	_____	_____

29a.   (ASK OF ALL RESPONDENTS) As you know, I've been keeping a list of the things that you say matter to you so far as where you choose to go for medical care. I'm going to be asking you some questions about these reasons that you've given, and it will be easier for you to answer if I write these reasons down for you on this card. (TRANSCRIBE REASONS FROM MASTER SHEET TO CARD, INFORMING THE RE-SPONDENT AS TO WHAT YOU ARE WRITING ON THE CARD AS YOU GO ALONG. BEFORE HANDING CARD TO RESPONDENT ASK) Are there any other things that matter to you in choosing where to go for ordinary, routine medical care that aren't on this list? (IF "YES", ADD THESE REASONS TO BOTH THE MASTER SHEET AND THE CARD)

Now, of the things listed on this card, which one matters the most to you in connection with where you go for your own general medical care? (RECORD "1" IN GENERAL "RANK-ORDER" COLUMN AND "10" IN GENERAL "IMPORTANCE" COLUMN OPPOSITE THE REASON SELECTED,

HAND RESPONDENT CARD "D", AND SAY:) Let's think in terms of a "1 - 10" scale and let's give __(reason ranked #1)__ a value of "10" which means "matters the most" on the scale on this card. Now I'd like you to give me numbers, from "1" through "9", which best describe how much each of the other reasons matter to you as far as choosing where you personally go for your own general medical care. If a reason matters almost as much as __(reason ranked #1)__ you would probably score it "8" or "9". If it matters only about half as much, you'd probably score it "5" or "6"; if it matters very little, you'd probably score it "2" or "3", and so forth. O.K., what score would you give to __(first unranked reason)__ ? (RECORD SCORE IN GENERAL "IMPORTANCE" COLUMN OPPOSITE THE REASON INVOLVED, AND CONTINUE THIS PROCEDURE UNTIL YOU HAVE OBTAINED SCORES FOR ALL REASONS. THEN, BEFORE ASKING THE NEXT PART OF THIS QUESTION, DIRECT YOUR ATTENTION TO THE GENERAL "RANK-ORDER" COLUMN IN WHICH YOU HAVE ALREADY ENTERED A "1" OPPOSITE THE REASON SCORED "10". IN THIS COLUMN RECORD A "2" FOR THE REASON WITH THE SECOND HIGHEST SCORE, A "3" FOR THE REASON WITH THE THIRD HIGHEST SCORE, ETC., UNTIL THE FIVE TOP REASONS HAVE BEEN SO RANKED. IN THE CASE OF TIES, ASSIGN THE SAME RANK, BUT IF TWO REASONS ARE TIED FOR SECOND PLACE, FOR INSTANCE, THE NEXT HIGHEST SCORE SHOULD BE RANKED "4" NOT "3".)

ONCE YOU HAVE DONE THIS, REFER RESPONDENT TO CARD "A" AND DIRECT YOUR ATTENTION TO THE FIVE SETS OF "YES-NO" BOXES ON THE MASTER SHEET FOR THE FIVE PLACES LISTED ON CARD "A". FOR EACH PLACE NOT ALREADY CHECKED "YES" SAY:) You say you have never gone to a _____. From what you may have seen, read or

heard about _____s, do you feel you know enough about them
to be able to say how satisfied you would be with certain things
about them? (CHECK THE APPROPRIATE "YES-NO" BOX FOR EACH PLACE
INVOLVED. IF 2 OR MORE PLACES ARE CHECKED "YES", CONTINUE; OTHER-
WISE, SKIP TO #29b, 29c, 30a OR 34a, WHICHEVER APPLIES.

You have said that (reason ranked #1) matters the most to you.
As far as (reason ranked #1) is concerned, which of the places
listed on Card "A" that you've had experience with or feel you know
enough about, do you think you would be most satisfied with as a
place to go for your own general medical care? (RECORD "10" UNDER
THIS PLACE IN THE GENERAL "SATISFACTION" COLUMNS OPPOSITE THIS
REASON AND HAND RESPONDENT CARD "E".) Let's think in terms of a
"1 - 10" scale again and let's give (place just mentioned) a score
of "10" as far as (reason ranked #1) is concerned. This means
"satisfied most" on the scale on this card. On the same basis as
before, what score would you give (first unscored place checked "Yes")
to indicate how satisfied you feel you would be with it as
far as (reason ranked #1) is concerned? What about
 (second unscored place checked "YES") ? (REPEAT FOR REMAINING
UNSCORED PLACES CHECKED "YES", ENTERING THE SCORES GIVEN FOR THE
VARIOUS PLACES IN THE APPROPRIATE COLUMNS, AND THEN REPEAT THE
ENTIRE PROCEDURE FOR THE REASONS RANKED SECOND, THIRD, FOURTH
AND FIFTH IN IMPORTANCE.)

29b.   (ASK ONLY OF THOSE FEMALE RESPONDENTS FOR WHOM "FEMALE PROBLEMS"
        HAS BEEN CHECKED "YES" ON THE MASTER SHEET) THE QUESTIONING
        WILL BE THE SAME AS IN #29a WITH THREE EXCEPTIONS:

1. THE REFERENCE WILL ALWAYS BE TO "THE MEDICAL TREATMENT OF
   FEMALE PROBLEMS" RATHER THAN TO "YOUR OWN GENERAL MEDICAL
   CARE", AND ALL SCORES WILL BE RECORDED IN THE "FEMALE
   PROBLEMS" COLUMNS ON THE MASTER SHEET.

2. THE QUESTIONING WILL NOT INVOLVE WRITING ANOTHER CARD AND
   WILL BEGIN BY HAVING THE RESPONDENT REFER TO THE PREVIOUSLY
   USED HAND-WRITTEN CARD AND ASKING HER WHICH ONE REASON MAT-
   TERS THE MOST ....

3. PRIOR TO DETERMINING "SATISFACTION SCORES" IT WILL NOT BE
   NECESSARY TO DETERMINE WHICH PLACES RESPONDENTS FEEL THEY
   KNOW ENOUGH ABOUT TO ANSWER. YOU WILL BE OBTAINING
   "SATISFACTION SCORES" FOR THE SAME PLACES AS IN #29a, SKIP-
   PING THIS SECTION ENTIRELY IF 2 OR MORE PLACES HAVE NOT BEEN
   CHECKED "YES".

29c. (ASK ONLY OF THOSE RESPONDENTS FOR WHOM "CHILDREN" HAS BEEN
      CHECKED "YES" ON THE MASTER SHEET) THE QUESTIONING WILL BE THE
      SAME AS IN #29b WITH ONE EXCEPTION:

      1. THE REFERENCE WILL ALWAYS BE TO "YOUR CHILD'S/CHILDREN'S
         MEDICAL CARE" RATHER THAN TO "THE MEDICAL TREATMENT OF
         FEMALE PROBLEMS", AND ALL SCORES WILL BE RECORDED IN THE
         "CHILDREN" COLUMNS ON THE MASTER SHEET.

30a. Now, to get back to your (child/children) if (he/she/one of your
      children) suddenly needed medical help at night or on Sunday, what
      would you or some other member of your household do?

      _____

      _____

      _____

b.   Suppose you wanted to reach your (child's/children's) doctor on
      the phone in the evening or on Sunday, how much trouble do you
      think you would have--a great deal, some, or no trouble at all?

                    Great Deal 1

                    Some 3

                    No Trouble At All 5

                    Don't Know 8

31a. Suppose you wanted your (child's/children's) doctor to come to
      your home to see the child at night or on a Sunday, how much
      trouble do you think there would be getting him to come--a
      great deal, some, or no trouble at all?

                    Great Deal 1

                    Some 3

                    No Trouble At All 5

                    Don't Know 8

b.   Suppose you simply wanted to bring your (child/children) to see
      a doctor--not have him come to your home--and you were willing to
      go where he asked. How much trouble do you think there would be
      seeing a doctor at night or on Sunday--a great deal, some, or no
      trouble at all?

                    Great Deal 1

                    Some 3

                    No Trouble At All 5

                    Don't Know 8

32a. Suppose you needed help for your (child/children) and decided to
      go to a Hospital Emergency Department. Which Hospital Emergency
      Department would you go to? _____

b.   Why would you go there? _____

_____

_____

_____

33a. Would you say your (child's/children's) health, in general, is ex-

cellent, good, fair, or poor?

           Excellent 1

           Good 3

           Fair 5

           Poor 7

           Don't Know 8

b.   When your children are your age, do you think their health will

be excellent, good, fair, or poor?

           Excellent 1

           Good 3

           Fair 5

           Poor 7

           Don't Know 8

c.   How about their children--do you think their children's health

will be excellent, good, fair, or poor?

           Excellent 1

           Good 3

           Fair 5

           Poor 7

           Don't Know 8

34a. Now we'd like to ask you some questions about how you would go

about getting help if you yourself suddenly needed medical help

at night or on a Sunday. What would you do?

b. If you wanted to reach your doctor on the phone at night or on
    Sunday, how much trouble do you think you would have--a great
    deal, some, or no trouble at all?

                Great Deal 1

                Some 3

                No Trouble At All 5

                Don't Know 8

c. Suppose you were sick and wanted a doctor to come to your house
    to examine you at night or on Sunday. How much trouble do you
    think you would have getting your doctor to come to your house--
    a great deal, some, or no trouble at all?

                Great Deal 1

                Some 3

                No Trouble At All 5

                Don't Know 8

d. Suppose you simply wanted to see your doctor--not have him come
    to your home--and you were willing to go where he asked. How
    much trouble do you think you would have seeing your doctor at
    night or on Sunday--a great deal, some, or no trouble at all?

                Great Deal 1

                Some 3

                No Trouble At All 5

                Don't Know 8

35a. Suppose you needed help and decided to go to a Hospital Emergency
      Department. Which Hospital Emergency Department would you go to?

b.   Why would you go there? _____

_____

_____

36a.   At the place where you usually go for medical care, how long do
       you usually have to wait to see a doctor?

       _____

b.   Does that seem like a reasonable amount of time, or is it too
     long to have to wait?

                    Reasonable 1

                    Too Long 5

                    Don't Know 8

c.   Do you usually make an appointment for a particular time when you
     go for medical care, do you simply stop in during the hours that
     they are open, or have you done both?

                    Usually make an appointment 1

                    Simply stop in 3

                    Have done both 5

                    Don't Know 8

37a.   Sometimes people become annoyed or even angered about things that
       happen to them when they go for health care. I mean not only
       medical treatment, but also the way they are treated as persons.
       Has this ever happened to you?

                    Yes 1

                    No 5   (SKIP TO #40a)

                    Don't Know 8   (SKIP TO #40a)

37b.   How often does it happen--frequently, occasionally, or has it
       happened only once?

                    Frequently 1

Occasionally 3

Only Once 5

NOTE: IF "FREQUENTLY" OR "OCCASIONALLY", ASK RESPONDENT TO

THINK OF THE INCIDENT WHICH ANNOYED OR ANGERED THEM MOST.

38a.   When did this incident occur? Was it:

Within the past six months, ... 1

6 months to a year ago, ... 3

1 to 5 years ago, or 5

Five years ago or longer? 7

b.   Where did the incident occur? Was it:

In Rochester, or 1

Somewhere else? 5

c.   Was it at a:

Hospital Emergency Room 1

Hospital Clinic 2

Private Doctor's Office 3

Clinic at Work, or 4

Neighborhood Health Center 5

d.   Who was the cause of the incident? Was it a:

Doctor 1

Nurse 3

Receptionist 5

Somebody Else 7

39a.   Please describe for me, briefly, what happened. _____

_____ _____

_____

_____

_____

b.   Were you annoyed or angered enough by this incident to cause you to change to another place for medical care?

```
Yes    1

No     5
```

40a.   Would you say your own health, in general, is excellent, good, fair, or poor?

```
Excellent ........  1

Good ............  3

Fair ............  5

Poor ............  7

Don't Know ........  8
```

b.   Are you married?

```
Yes    1

No     5   (SKIP TO #41a)
```

c.   What about the health of your spouse? Would you say it is excellent, good, fair, or poor?

```
Excellent ........  1

Good ............  3

Fair ............  5

Poor ............  7

Don't Know ........  8
```

41a.   Do you think about your health fairly often, once in a while, or hardly ever? (CHECK UNDER "a" BELOW)

b.   Do you talk about your health with your family and friends fairly often, once in a while, or hardly ever? (CHECK UNDER "b" BELOW)

	"a"	"b"
	Think About	Talk About
Fairly Often	1	1

Once in a While	3	3
Hardly Ever	5	5
Don't Know ....,	8	8

42a. Do you see a doctor for regular check-ups, even when you're feeling all right?

Yes   1

No   5   (SKIP TO #43)

b. How frequently? _____

43a. People frequently call or visit a doctor about medical problems which, though routine to the doctor, are often of considerable concern to the individual. To accommodate the needs of these people, some doctors now use what are known as para-professionals - medical personnel with special training and experience, who in some specialized areas are better able to serve the patient than is the doctor himself. They are qualified to treat many of the routine problems that people have, and they relieve the doctor of many of the tasks that don't require the greater expertise of the doctor. At the same time they help to ensure that the doctor can see more quickly those patients that do need his attention. In summary, the purpose of para-medical personnel is to enable the doctor to treat his patients more efficiently and to save patients from perhaps unnecessary trips to his office. We'd like to know how willing you would be to see such a person in such instances instead of your doctor. Would you be very willing, would you have doubts, or wouldn't you be willing at all?

Very Willing 1

Would Have Doubts 3

Not Willing At All 5

Don't Know 8

b. If such a person were to be made available for telephone consultation after normal working hours, is there considerable, some,
a little, or no chance that you would call him rather than the
doctor, should the need arise?

> Considerable 1
>
> Some 3
>
> A Little 5
>
> No Chance 7
>
> Don't Know 8

44a. The next few questions have to do with the responsibility for
planning and control of health care in our country. Some people
say that the planning and control of health care decisions should
be made by doctors and other members of the health professions.
Others say that the people who use health services should have
more of a say in these decisions. Please tell me how you feel
about this question. (HAND RESPONDENT CARD "F") Please tell me
the number on this card that best represents how you feel?
Planning and control of health care decision should be made:

1. Exclusively by doctors and other professionals

2. In the main by doctors and other professionals

3. More by doctors and other professionals

4. Equally by doctors/professionals and by the people who use
    health services

5. More by the people who use health services

6. In the main by the people who use health services

7. Exclusively by the people who use health services

44b. There is much concern about the rapid rise in medical and hospital
costs. Some feel there should be a government health insurance

plan which would cover all medical and hospital expenses. Others feel that medical expenses should be paid by individuals and through private insurance like Blue Cross. (HAND RESPONDENT CARD "G") If "1" represents the position that there should be a government health insurance plan and "7" represents the position that medical expenses should be paid by individuals through private insurance plans, which of the seven numbers on this card best represents your opinion on this matter?

Government Health   Paid by Individuals
Insurance Plan   1   2   3   4   5   6   7   Through Private Insurance

c. Which of these numbers do you feel best represents the opinion of the Democratic party on this matter?

Government Health   Paid by Individuals
Insurance Plan   1   2   3   4   5   6   7   Through Private Insurance

d. Which do you feel best represents the opinion of the Republican party?

Government Health   Paid by Individuals
Insurance Plan   1   2   3   4   5   6   7   Through Private Insurance

e. What do you think is the most important problem in the area of medical care that the government should do something about?

_____

_____

_____

f. How important do you think this problem is--the most important problem facing the government, very important, not so important, or not important at all?

                Most Important Problem 1

                Very Important Problem 3

Not So Important 5

Not Important At All 7

No Opinion 8

g.   Which political party do you think is most likely to do what you want on this issue, the Republicans or the Democrats?

Republicans 1

Democrats 3

No Difference 5

Neither 7

No Opinion 8

45a.   How many adults, 18 years of age or older, including yourself, are living in this household at the present time?

_____

b.   And you have already told me there (are/is) _____ (children/child) under 18. (NOTE: IF "0" TO #45b, SKIP TO #46c)

c.   (IF "1" TO #45b) What is his/her age? _____ ____

d.   (IF "2" TO #45b) What are their ages? _____ _____

e.   (IF "3" OR MORE TO #45b) What is the age of the oldest? _____
What is the age of the youngest? _____

46a.   Do you think your children, when they get older and have their own families, will be more satisfied with life in general, about equally satisfied, or less satisfied than you are at the present time?

More 1

Equally 3

Less 5

Don't Know 8

46b. Do you expect that the (child/children) under 18 living in your household now will go to college?

           Yes 1

           No 5

           Don't Know 8

c. How important do you think it is these days for young people to complete four years of college? Is it:

           Absolutely Necessary 1

           Very Important 3

           Somewhat Important, or 5

           Not Important At All 7

           Don't Know 8

47a. Are you more satisfied with life in general, about equally satisfied, or less satisfied now than when you were growing up?

           More 1

           Equally 3

           Less 5

           Don't Know 8

b. When you were growing up, would you say your family was pretty well off financially, about average, or did they have trouble making ends meet?

           Well Off 1

           About Average 3

           Had Trouble 5

           Don't Know 8

c.   Would you say you are better off, about the same, or not as
well off financially now as your family was when you were growing
up?

```
                  Better ............  1

                  Same .............  3

                  Not As Well Off ...  5

                  Don't Know ........  8
```

48a.   In what year were you born?   _____

b.   Were you born in the United States?

```
        Yes    1   (ASK #48c AND SKIP TO #49a)

        No     5   (SKIP TO #48d)
```

c.   In what state?   _____

d.   In what country were you born?   _____

49a.   Did you grow up in the United States?

```
        Yes    1   (ASK #49b AND SKIP TO #49d)

        No     5   (SKIP TO #49c)
```

b.   In what state or states?   _____ __

c.   In what country did you grow up?   _____ __

d.   Were you brought up mostly:

```
                  On a farm ...........  1

                  In a small town ......  3

                  In a small city ......  5

                  In a large city ......  7
```

50a.   Do you own your own home, rent, or have some other arrangement?

```
                  Own .............  1   (SKIP TO #51a)

                  Rent ............  3   (SKIP TO #51a)

                  Other Arrangement.  5
```

b.   What type of arrangement do you have? _____

_____

51a.   Do you have any type of health or medical insurance?

Yes   1

No   5   (SKIP TO #51d)

b.   What type do you have--Blue Cross/Blue Shield, Medicare, Medicaid,

or some other type?

Blue Cross/Blue Shield 1   (SKIP TO #51d)

Medicare 3   (SKIP TO #51d)

Medicaid 5   (SKIP TO #51d)

Other Type 7

c.   What other type do you have? _____

d.   How do you usually pay for medical services not covered by insur-

ance--do you pay cash or charge them?

Pay Cash 1

Charge 3

Both 5

52a.   Are you currently employed full-time, employed part-time, retired,

unemployed, (or) a full-time student, (or) (FEMALE RESPONDENTS ONLY)

a housewife?

Employed Full-Time 1

Employed Part-Time 2

Retired 3

Unemployed 4

Full-Time Student 5   (SKIP TO #52d)

Housewife 6   (SKIP TO #52d)

b.   Where (do/did) you work? _____

c.   What type of work (do/did) you do? _____ _____

d.   Are you the head of the household?

                Yes   1   (SKIP TO #52i)

                No   5

e.   What is your relationship to the head of the house? _____

f.   Is the person who is the head of this household employed full-time,

     employed part-time, retired, unemployed, or a full-time student?

                Employed Full-Time 1

                Employed Part-Time 2

                Retired 3

                Unemployed 4

                Full-Time Student 5   (SKIP TO #52i)

g.   Where (does/did) this person work? _____

h.   What type of work (does/did) this person do? _____

i.   What type of work did the head of the household you grew up in do?

        _____

53.   (HAND RESPONDENT CARD "H") Which of these best describes your

     marital status?

                Married - Living with Husband or Wife 1

                Married - Spouse in Service 2

                Separated ..., ... 3

                Divorced 4

                Widow/Widower 5

                Single 6

                Single - Living with Common Law Spouse 7

54a. (HAND RESPONDENT CARD "I") Which of these best describes how far

     you went in school? (CHECK UNDER "a" BELOW)

b.   (IF "NO" TO #52d) Which best describes how far the head of the

house went in school?   (CHECK UNDER "b" BELOW)

	"a"	"b"
Did Not Attend School	1	1
Attended Grammar School	2	2
Completed Grammar School	3	3
Attended High School	4	4
Graduated from High School	5	5
Attended College	6	6
Graduated from College	7	7
Have Done Graduate Work	8	8
Have a Graduate Degree	9	9

55b.   Do you consider yourself a Protestant, a Catholic, a Jew or a

member of some other religious faith?

Protestant 1

Catholic 2   (SKIP TO #56a)

Jew 3   (SKIP TO #56a)

Other 4   (SKIP TO #56a)

No Answer 9   (SKIP TO #56a)

b.   What denomination is that - Baptist, Methodist, Presbyterian?

_____

56a.   Generally speaking, do you usually think of yourself as a

Republican, a Democrat, an Independent, or something else?

Republican 1

Democrat 3

Independent 5

Something Else 7

No Preference 8

b.   (IF "REPUBLICAN" OR "DEMOCRAT") Would you call yourself a strong

                    _____, or a not very strong _____?

                         Strong Republican 1

                         Not Very Strong

                             Republican 3

                         Strong Democrat 5

                         Not Very Strong

                             Democrat 7

                         Not Sure 8

c.   (IF "INDEPENDENT" , "SOMETHING ELSE", "NO PREFERENCE") Do you

     usually think of yourself as closer to the Republican or to the

     Democrat party?

                         Republican 1

                         Democratic 3

                         Neither 5

                         Don't Know 8

57a. (HAND RESPONDENT CARD "J") Which of these categories comes closet

     to your estimate of what the total income of all the members of

     your household will be this year. Income includes salary, wages,

     pension, Social Security, welfare, and any other income before

     taxes.

                         Under $2,500 0

                         $2,500 - $4,999 1

                         $5,000 - $7,499 2

                         $7,500 - $9,999 3

                         $10,000 - $12,499 4

                         $12,500 - $14,999 5

                         $15,000 - $17,499 6

$17,500 - $19,999 7

$20,000 or over 8

Don't Know/Refused 9

b. About what percent of this total is represented by the income of
    the head of the house?   _____%

Respondent _____

Address _____

City or Town _____

Sex: Male   (__)   Female   (__)

Race: White (__)   Black (__)   Other   (__)

Spanish-Speaking Ethnic Background? Yes (__)   No (__)

Time Interview Completed: _____

Interviewer's Initials _____ Date _____

Validated _____ Edited _____

MASTER SHEET

		Yes	No
Record below the reasons that relate	Hospital Emergency Room	(_)	(_)
to the respondent's choice or use of	Hospital Clinic	(_)	(_)
different health facilities, indicating	Private Doctor's Office	(_)	(_)
which question(s) the reasons relate to.	Clinic at Work	(_)	(_)
	Neighborhood Health Center	(_)	(_)

Reason: CODE _____
                                                     QUEST.

Reason: CODE _____
       QUEST.

Reason: CODE _____
       QUEST.

Reason: CODE _____

Reason: CODE _____
       QUEST.

Reason: CODE _____
       QUEST.

Reason: CODE _____
       QUEST.

Reason: CODE _____
       QUEST.

Reason: CODE _____
       QUEST.

Reason: CODE _____
       QUEST.

GENERAL		FEMALE PROBLEMS		CHILDREN	
Yes ( ) No ( )		Yes ( ) No ( )		Yes ( ) No ( )	

RANK-ORDER	IMPORTANCE	SATISFACTION							RANK-ORDER	IMPORTANCE	SATISFACTION							RANK-ORDER	IMPORTANCE	SATISFACTION						
		HOSP. E.R.	HOSP. CLIN.	PVT. DR.	AT WORK		NHC				HOSP. E.R.	HOSP. CLIN.	PVT. DR.	AT WORK		NHC					HOSP. E.R.	HOSP. CLIN.	PVT. DR.	AT WORK		NHC

Index

About the Authors

William C. Stratmann is a consultant on health-care systems. He received the Ph.D. in political science from the University of Rochester and has held appointments at the State University of New York College at Brockport, the University of Vermont, and the University of Rochester. His current interest is in the development of computerized information systems for clinical care, education, and research.

Ralph Ullman is an assistant professor of public health at Columbia University. He received the bachelor's degree from Cornell University and master's degrees in business administration and community health from the University of Rochester. Currently, he is a candidate for the Ph.D. in public policy analysis from the University of Pennsylvania. His doctoral dissertation examines aspects of health maintenance organization enrollment and national health insurance.